OXFORD MEDICAL PUBLICATIONS

Breast cancer

THE FACTS

Breast cancer

THE FACTS

MICHAEL BAUM

Professor of Surgery
King's College Hospital

with a chapter by
Sylvia Denton

Nurse-Counsellor
Department of Surgery, King's College Hospital

OXFORD
OXFORD UNIVERSITY PRESS
NEW YORK TORONTO
1981

Oxford University Press, Walton Street, Oxford OX2 6DP

London Glasgow New York Toronto
Delhi Bombay Calcutta Madras Marachi
Kuala Lumpur Singapore Hong Kong Tokyo
Nairobi Dar es Salaam Cape Town
Melbourne Wellington
and associate companies in
Beirut Berlin Ibadan Mexico City

British Library Cataloguing in Publication Data

Baum, Michael
    Breast cancer. – (Oxford medical publications)
    1. Breast – Cancer
    I. Title
    616.99'4'49   RC280.B8
    ISBN 0-19-261265-4

Typeset by Hope Services, Abingdon
Printed in Great Britain by
R. Clay & Co. Ltd., Bungay

THIS BOOK IS DEDICATED TO THE MEMORY OF
MY DEAR PARENTS
MARY AND ISIDOR BAUM

Preface

When I first started to write this book, I thought it might end up competing for entry into the list of the shortest books ever published. Although one could write an extremely long book on breast cancer, padded out with a variety of strongly held and contradictory opinion, dogma, or emotional rhetoric, all this would merely cloud the truth of the profundity of our ignorance concerning breast cancer.

What are facts? The *Oxford English Dictionary* defines a fact as a datum of experience, and certainly with carcinoma of the breast there are plenty of such data. Unfortunately, clinical experience in itself is not sufficient, as we often interpret our experiences in the light of pre-existing hypothetical biological models. If I admit right from the outset that we do not even know the natural course of untreated early breast cancer, then the reader will be able to judge just how shaky are the foundations upon which we have to build our knowledge of this disease. For obvious reasons, medical authors writing for the lay public tend to be embarrassed about exposing their nakedness, whereas books or magazine articles written by most journalists on the subject tend to sensationalize the subject, describing non-existent 'breakthroughs' with the occasional sprinkling of sexual titillation. In addition, books and articles on breast cancer written by members of the feminist lobby are beginning to appear on both sides of the Atlantic. The characteristic theme of these tracts is the right of the woman to choose her own treatment. It is my opinion that this latter group of authors or journalists will probably prove to be as damaging to progress as the older type of reactionary surgeon who was content unthinkingly to carry out radical mastectomies for decade after decade.

Preface

Members of the feminist lobby claim that they already know all the answers to the questions that I am trying to pose in this book. For example, they *know* that breast conservation is a safe alternative to mastectomy (but it is highly unlikely that two such extremely different treatments should ultimately have identical outcomes). To date, there is no information as to the exact risk entailed by the conservative approach. Therefore, the militant feminist could be doing her sisters untold harm by promoting therapeutic anarchy and perpetuation of our ignorance on the subject.

Perhaps it should be emphasized that, contrary to their stereotype, surgeons do not lack compassion, and are motivated by care and concern for their patients; apart from the odd maverick financial profit does not enter into the equation. It is my impression that in the United States there exists an irrational mood of anti-professionalism associated with a profound distrust of the motives of American surgeons that has led to a new cottage industry of second and third opinions. I hope that this book will contribute in a small way to the prevention of spread of these unhelpful attitudes.

It is the intention of this book to cater for an intelligent lay public, and also for the paramedical professional groups and the general practitioner, who so often has to pick up the pieces once a patient and her family hear that the diagnosis is breast cancer. In addition, I would hope that this book would help women on both sides of the Atlantic to collaborate with their physicians when treatment options are discussed. I believe that the current status of 'informed consent' is a ruse to protect the doctors from rapacious lawyers and litigious patients rather than to protect the patient herself. On the one hand, short of taking a five-year medical course, no woman can truly be informed about her disease and its treatment; but on the other hand, the need for the legal formula surely indicates a loss of trust between the public and the medical profession. Perhaps this book, in which the facts are laid out side by side with our areas of ignorance,

Preface

in an open and honest way, will contribute to a small extent to the regeneration of trust between the client and the professional.

At a recent international surgical conference in the United States of America I was trying to express this point of view. At the end of my talk I was having to field a barrage of hostile questioning from the surgeons in the audience. Most of them wanted me to come off the fence and to define exactly how I would advocate the treatment of early breast cancer. Contrary to what they thought, I was not holding any secrets back when I said that I truly did not know the right answers but I felt confident that I knew the right questions. After all that is what science is about: the framing of the right questions so that we constantly approximate to the truth, corroborating or refuting our hypotheses and thus establishing what are true facts. The doctor and the patient are equal partners in this search for the truth, which can progress only by the rigorous application of the scientific method. As will be seen in this book, scientific method is not incompatible with true compassion. I truly believe that the surgeons, physicians, radiotherapists, medical oncologists, and other health professionals who are dedicating their lives to the scientific evaluation of therapy for breast cancer care far more for womankind than their self-appointed custodians.

London   MB
April 1981

Contents

1

The history of breast cancer

Over 12 000 women die of breast cancer every year in the United Kingdom; in the United States of America the figure is 34 000. It ranks as the commonest cancer in women and the commonest cause of death amongst women in the 35–55 age group. Any individual woman in her lifetime stands a 1 in 14 chance of developing the disease, and there is even some evidence that the annual incidence and mortality rates are increasing throughout the Western Hemisphere. Because of these disturbing facts the subject has become highly charged and emotional, so much so as to cloud rational discussion. Television, newspapers, and women's journals commonly seize on the subject with the expressed desire to inform the public, but in a way that the cynic may suspect is designed to improve programme ratings or newspaper circulation. As a result of all this publicity a lay person could be excused from believing that the disease is a new one, whereas in fact it is probably as ancient as womankind.

Cancer of the breast has been recognized as an entity since the times of the ancient Egyptians. An early papyrus describes how it is differentiated from mastitis. No treatment was advocated other than cautery for the ulcerated tumour. Surgery for breast cancer was practised by the ancient Greeks, but Hypocrates considered no treatment at all was superior to surgery: probably a very wise opinion in those days. In Rome at the time of Celsus, a prototype of radical mastectomy (total removal of the breast) was probably being performed. This can be deduced from the fact that Celsus in an ancient text advises against the removal of certain muscles at the time of amputation of the breast. In some ways he also distinguished between early and advanced disease, recognizing

1

the futility of surgery in the latter. One shudders to think of the suffering of these poor women in the days before anaes- thesia and antisepsis, and the so-called Dark Ages must have produced a welcome respite from the surgeon's amputation knife. According to the doctrines of Galen, who dominated medical thinking between the classical period and the Renais- sance, melancholia (black bile) was the causal factor in the development of breast cancer and special diets designed to avoid the accumulation of black bile were recommended. In addition, exorcism plus a variety of topical applications, often of an unspeakable nature, were commonplace. It is perhaps salutary to remember that during the third century A.D. mas- tectomy was reserved as a punitive rather than a therapeutic weapon and poor Saint Agatha, the patron saint of the breast, was sent to her untimely grave following bilateral amputation of her breasts.

During the Renaissance, Vesalius and Fabricus again rec- ommended mastectomy, with a wide surgical excision of the tumour, but in addition they advocated ligatures to control the bleeding rather than cautery. LeDran (1685–1770) recog- nized that the disease spread to the regional lymph nodes in the armpit (axillary nodes) and advocated that they were removed if enlarged. He was probably the first to describe the poor outlook associated with involvement of the lymph nodes, a clinical observation of far-reaching importance, on the basis of which modern clinicians are selecting patients for trials of drug therapy following mastectomy (see Chapter 7). Petit (1674–1750) advocated removal of the primary growth and the axillary nodes in continuity with it.

It is difficult to judge the success rate of these procedures because of the absence of formally collected statistics of recurrence rates and survival. However, there is anecdotal evidence that some women survived these operations per- formed under such primitive circumstances and went on to enjoy a normal expectation of life. I have recently had drawn to my attention a charming example of such an event occurring

The history of breast cancer

in L'Hôtel Dieu, Quebec, the oldest hospital in North America. In 1700 Sister Barbier de l'Assomption developed a breast tumour whilst working as a nurse for the famous surgeon Michel Sarazan at L'Hôtel Dieu. Putting herself in the hands of God first, and surgeon second, she submitted to mastectomy, made an uneventful recovery, and did not die until thirty years later, by which time she had risen in the ranks to Mother Superior.

In the middle part of the last century surgeons started to keep reasonable records of their experience treating breast cancer, and Sir James Paget's experience (1853) of 74 cases treated by mastectomy with 100 per cent recurrence rate within eight years is probably fairly typical of that era. In 1842 James Syme, writing in his textbook *Principles of surgery*, stated: 'It appears that the results of operations for carcinoma when the glands are affected is almost always unsatisfactory, however perfectly they may seem to have been taken away. The reason of [*sic*] this probably is that the glands do not participate in the disease unless the system is strongly disposed to it, and consequently their removal, however freely and effectively executed, cannot prevent the patients' relapse'. These are highly significant comments: first, they reflect that some form of radical operations were being carried out in an attempt to 'perfectly take away' the affected glands, and, secondly, it again illustrates the ineluctable truth, first noted by LeDran, that significant involvement of the axillary nodes is indicative or symptomatic of what is already a *systemic* disease – in other words, the disease is beginning to affect other parts of the body. It has taken well over 100 years to recognize the wisdom of Sir James Syme. In spite of his observations surgeons persisted in their attempts to clear the axilla 'perfectly'. Thus Banks (1878) advocated routine removal of axillary nodes, as he recognized that even impalpable nodes contain tumour on occasions. So it would appear that prior to Halsted's description of the radical mastectomy in the 1890s, surgeons were already carrying out routine removal of the axillary nodes, in addition to removing the breast with or without the pectoral musculature.

It is, therefore, of great historical importance to consider the results of treatment for breast cancer in the period immediately prior to 1890 in order to determine exactly what impact Halsted had on the management of breast cancer, particularly as the 'Halsted radical procedure' still remains conventional therapy in many parts of the world today. In 1880 Gross published a treatise on the treatment of tumours of the mammary gland. This elegantly written book receives scant attention in most literature on the subject of breast cancer, yet it provides a beautifully clear insight into the status of the disease in the immediate pre-Halsted era, and should perhaps be considered as a baseline on which to judge the validity of the classical radical mastectomy.

From the outset it must be recognized that the progression, or staging, of the disease had not been described and most operations were being carried out for locally advanced cancers rather than the small breast lumps which are the common presentation of the disease today. This fact is clearly demonstrated by the following statistics. Gross described a series of 660 cases, 70 per cent of whom had skin infiltration on presentation, and in 25 per cent skin ulceration was present. Two-thirds of the cases had obviously-involved axillary nodes, and a third of the cases had palpable supraclavicular nodes (see page 19). Five hundred and nineteen cases were operated upon, somewhat more than half being treated by simple (total) mastectomy, and the rest with a simple mastectomy plus some form of axillary clearance. There were 17 per cent operative deaths, 80 per cent local recurrences, and 9 per cent survived ten years. From post mortem studies, he demonstrated that one in eight cases had secondary tumours (metastases) in bone, without glandular involvement, and even postulated that the spread of the disease was via the bloodstream rather than the lymphatic system. From similar studies he noted that nodes removed because they were thought to be involved with tumour often showed benign changes, and that all such patients went on to survive for more than six years. These are truly remarkable observations which, again, have been rediscovered within the last 20 years, and form the basis of the contemporary biological model that describes the behaviour of breast cancer.

On referring to Halsted's early publications concerning the results of the radical mastectomy, one reads of a high proportion of three-year 'cures'. His criteria for a 'cure' would not be acceptable by today's standards. To get a true perspective of the long-term outcome of his methods of treatment it is necessary to consult the records of the Johns Hopkins Hospital in Baltimore between 1889 and 1931. During this period nearly 900 patients were operated upon by Halsted or his students. Six per cent of patients died soon after their operation, and the local recurrence rate was 30 per cent, but the very disappointing ten-year survival rate was 12 per cent. So it can be seen that at the turn of the century the introduction of the radical procedure improved upon local control of the disease without influencing long-term survival.

Between the early 1930s and the 1950s there were apparent improvements in the treatment of breast cancer, probably resulting from the interaction of many factors. For example, earlier presentation of the disease due to better health education, or the loss of false modesty that characterized the Victorian age, may have played their part. These considerations aside, there is little doubt that the most important development that led to the improvement in survival following mastectomy was the development of clinical methods of classifying the stage of progression of the disease. Almost simultaneously in England and America two staging systems were developed which divided breast cancer up into different groups of patients with outlooks predicted on the basis of clearly defined clinical signs. In the early 1940s the Manchester staging system was described in England with Stages I and II representing the operable ('curable') groups of cases; Stage III the locally advanced disease where surgery was doomed to failure; and Stage IV the patient with obvious distant metastases. In 1943 Haagenson in America described the Columbia clinical classification with Stages A and B representing the operable group, and Stage C the locally advanced cases, where again surgery was doomed to failure. As a result, with better and better selection, the ten-year survival rates following mastectomy improved from about 10 per cent in the 1920s to about 50 per cent in the 1950s. This figure of a 50 per cent ten-year survival has remained stubbornly fixed until the time of writing, in spite of all the apparent benefits of early diagnosis, improved surgical techniques, and the use of postoperative radiotherapy. It is only within the last two or three years, with the exploitation of the clinical observations of Syme and Gross from over a century ago, that it looks as if significant inroads are being made into the mortality statistics of this commonest of all malignant diseases of women.

2

Risk factors and prevention

Introduction

If the causes of breast cancer were fully understood, then it might be conceivable to prevent the disease by the manipulation of life-style or by the identification and preventive treatment of the women most at risk. The two most promising lines of research in this respect are, first, the study of the geographical variation of the incidence of the disease and secondly, by the study of the risk factors acting within a given population.

Geographical variation

It has long been recognized that there are striking differences in the incidence of breast cancer in different geographical areas, and, in addition, there is also evidence that the natural progression of the disease is different within these areas. Until recently the most marked difference in incidence of breast cancer has been between the high rate in Western Europe and the United States of America and the extremely low rates in South East Asia. Over the last ten years there has been a suggestion that the rate for the disease amongst Japanese women has been climbing to that seen amongst expatriate Japanese living in the United States of America, where second-generation Japanese women experience the same risk as their American compatriots. Curiously, the incidence for Japanese women living in Hawaii appears to be midway between that in Japan and that found amongst the Japanese community in the USA. Furthermore, when the disease does develop in a Japanese woman it seems to run a more benign course, stage for stage, than might be expected in Western Europe.

In between these extremes it is possible to construct a league table of incidence (Table 1). The general impression one gets from studying this league table is that the more developed the countries in the Western sense of the word, the higher the risk. This finding, coupled with the suggestion that the incidence amongst Japanese women is creeping up as they develop the American way of life, forces one to assume that environmental factors act more powerfully than genes in determining which women will be most likely to develop the disease. Diet may be the first factor to spring to mind, but perhaps other cultural or behavioural patterns related to birth control and lactation could also be implicated. For example, the more under-developed the country, the earlier a woman has her first pregnancy. She is more likely to have a larger family than her Western counterpart and she is more likely to breast-feed than bottle-feed her babies.

Within a geographical area of overall high incidence, which would include the United Kingdom, sub-groups can readily be recognized now, in which the risk of developing breast cancer may vary from approximately half to two-fold that of the average risk in that region.

Lactation and childbearing

As milking cows virtually never develop carcinoma of the udders, breast-feeding was one of the first risk factors to be considered amongst women. Initial reports suggested that lactation did indeed have a protective effect on the development of carcinoma of the breast. More recently it has been demonstrated that child-bearing rather than lactation plays the protective role. Childless women over the age of 30 form the high-risk group, whereas women who have borne children at an early age, whether they have breast-fed or bottle-fed, seem to share the same degree of relative protection. There is

Risk factors and prevention

Table 1. *Annual death rate from breast cancer per 100 000 females at risk*

20–25	Netherlands
	England and Wales
	Denmark
	Scotland
	Canada
	New Zealand
	U.S.A.
	Ireland
	Israel
15–19	Australia
	Sweden
	France
	Italy
10–14	Finland
	Hungary
	Portugal
	Poland
5–9	Hong Kong
	Chile
	Greece
	Yugoslavia
Less than 5	Mexico
	China
	Japan
	Thailand

one unusually bizarre occurrence, which is perhaps contrary to the above generalization, that is to be found amongst the Hong Kong boat-women. These women suckle their children almost entirely on the left breast, partly because of the way their tunics open, and partly so as to leave their right hand free for rowing their boats. If they develop breast cancer it appears to be significantly more common in the right breast, which has perhaps been under-used.

The data concerning childbearing has been further refined to demonstrate that the age at first pregnancy carries the most important negative risk factor. Thus, women who have their first child under the age of 25 have about half the risk of women having their first child over the age of 30, or those who remain childless through life. It is worth noting that the first epidemiological study of carcinoma of the breast reported in the eighteenth century stated that a group of nuns living in a convent in France showed a high prevalence of breast cancer.

It has also been suggested that the number of menstrual cycles occurring before the first pregnancy may be the ultimate determinant, and this may further explain the difference in incidence of the disease between the developed and the developing countries. Thus, at one extreme the young English girl on a more than adequate diet will start menstruating at the age of 11 or 12 and will perhaps postpone pregnancy until over the age of 25 so as to pursue her own career, whereas her counterpart, an under-nourished Asian peasant girl, may not start menstruating until the age of 17 or 18, and will perhaps become pregnant at her second ovulation.

Administered hormones

Following on from the above, the obvious question is whether the contraceptive pill or hormone replacement therapy may increase the risk of the development of breast cancer. This is a reasonable question because of other indirect evidence that internal hormone levels may influence the development of the disease. It is known that women who have an artificial menopause before the age of 35 experience a lower risk. The annual incidence rates appear to dip during the years when women pass through the natural menopause, and there is a clearly established link between abnormal oestrogen levels and the incidence of breast cancer amongst men. Added to this is the fascinating and unique investigation by Bulbrook and Hayward who have studied prospectively the female population of the island of Guernsey. They collected samples of urine from all the women on the island and stored them in a cold room for later analysis. Whenever a woman developed

Risk factors and prevention

carcinoma of the breast, her urine was tested for various hormone metabolites and compared with that in a control group of urine samples. They were able to demonstrate that abnormalities in the excretion of hormone metabolites could be found up to ten years in advance of the women developing carcinoma of the breast.

To come back to the original question, therefore: is there any evidence that the contraceptive pill or hormone replacement therapy increases the risk of women developing breast cancer? As far as the first part of the question is concerned, the evidence so far is greatly reassuring. Several studies have failed to demonstrate any association with the taking of the pill and the subsequent development of breast cancer; on the contrary, one large prospective study conducted by the Royal College of General Practitioners in the United Kingdom has actually shown reduction in the incidence of benign breast disease. Finally, those women who do develop breast cancer, having been on the pill within a year or two of its development, appear to develop disease which carries a better outlook.

The question concerning the risks of hormone replacement therapy (HRT) for menopausal symptoms has yet to be answered satisfactorily. A number of studies have failed to demonstrate any correlation between HRT and the eventual development of breast cancer, but one large study reported from America has suggested that there is a slightly increased risk amongst women who have been taking HRT in excess of ten years. I can produce an interesting snippet of anecdotal evidence that might relate HRT to breast cancer. A woman came to my Breast Clinic with a large, locally advanced breast cancer. She had been prescribed HRT for severe menopausal symptoms 20 years before, and had continued on the oestrogen-containing tablets by repeat prescription ever since. In the first instance I merely advised her to stop taking the pills, and she had a complete regression of the disease that lasted for nine months before it eventually recurred.

Breast cancer: the facts

Genetic factors

Quite independent of parity, race, and diet, a family history of breast cancer must also be considered a risk factor. Thus a woman with any first-degree relative (mother, grandmother, sister, or daughter) who has developed carcinoma of the breast is herself at greater risk than a woman with no family history of breast cancer. These risks must not be exaggerated but at their most extreme there is a sub-group of women who have a near 50 per cent chance of developing carcinoma of the breast in their lifetime. These are women whose mothers developed bilateral breast cancer under the age of 35. As can be imagined, such women are a very rare group indeed, but it is now being suggested that perhaps subcutaneous mastectomy with sialastic implants might be advocated as a preventative measure for these *rara aves*.

Viruses

In certain strains of mice it is well recognized that breast cancer can be transmitted from mothers to daughters, which almost invariably develop carcinoma of the breast. If the female offspring are separated from the mothers and fed artificially or by foster-parents, the new generation fails to develop the disease. Analysis of the milk of these high incidence strains has demonstrated particles, referred to as the Bitner virus, which carry the enzyme reverse transcriptase known to be associated with carcinogenesis. There is no clear evidence from human studies that the disease can be transmitted by viruses in this vertical fashion, although one study amongst an isolated community of Iranian women who appear to have a one in five chance of developing breast cancer in their lifetime has demonstrated viral particles in the milk with similar characteristics to the Bitner virus. So far no prospective study has been published to compare the incidence rates amongst women who had either been breast-fed or bottle-fed at birth.

Risk factors and prevention

Ionizing radiation

Japanese women who were exposed to radiation following the atomic bomb attacks on Hiroshima and Nagasaki are still continuing to develop carcinoma of the breast at a higher rate than might be expected from the age-matched control population. The risk of developing these cancers appears to be directly related to the exposure they received as judged by their distance from the epicentre of the blasts at the time of the bombing. Other studies have demonstrated that women who received repeated chest X-rays during the treatment of tuberculosis are also at a higher risk of developing carcinoma of the breast. There seems little doubt, therefore, that ionizing radiation acting directly on the breast duct epithelium contributes to the development of carcinoma of the breast. It is not known at what dosage level the risk becomes insignificant, so there is a slight anxiety that repeated radiographs of the breast (mammograms) in screening programmes may produce accumulated doses of radiation to the breast that could induce cancer. However, this risk should not be exaggerated when compared with the possible benefits of a screening programme (see Chapter 6).

Miscellaneous risk factors

Many other associations have been described implicating environmental and genetic factors which, together with the previous discussions, can be summarized by a quotation from a delightful paper published by Doctors Leis and Raciti in 1976: 'The search for the patient with the highest risk of developing breast cancer would culminate in finding a 51-year-old, fat, hypothyroid Caucasian nun living in a cold climate in the Western Hemisphere, with a wet type of cerumen and a prolonged menstrual history, whose mother and sister had pre-menopausal bilateral breast cancer, who was nursed by a mother who had B viral particles in her milk, who has had endometrial cancer and a cancer in one breast,

13

whose random biopsy of the other breast showed a pre-cancerous mastopathy, who has a low estriol fraction, who is immuno-deficient, who received heavy radiation exposure during treatment for tuberculosis by repeated fluoroscopies, and who has a high dietary fat intake.' One feels that such a woman would be immediately recognizable!

Prevention

It can be seen from the above that there are many tantalizing clues to the aetiology of carcinoma of the breast. One can assume that the genetic factors cannot be controlled as a woman has little chance of choosing her parents, but the environmental factors which may indirectly produce changes in endogenous hormone levels that sensitize the lactiferous duct epithelium could perhaps be modulated. There is much clinical experimental work going on in the world at present with these aims in mind and I for one am reasonably optimistic that prevention is a realistic goal.

3

Structure and function of the breast

Embryological development

The breast develops in sixth week of foetal life. The mammary ducts develop by growing down from the skin surface through the layers of skin in a similar manner to the sweat glands. (It has even been suggested that the breasts are in fact modified sweat glands.) Very rarely the breast may fail to develop altogether on one side or the other and this congenital anomaly may be associated with absence of the shoulder muscles as well. Also rarely, a supernumerary breast may develop along the line of the so-called milk streak, which may be sufficiently well differentiated as to enlarge and lactate during pregnancy and the post-partum period. I personally have seen only one such example where a third breast had developed on one side, causing alarm to a young woman during the early weeks of her first pregnancy. There are many recorded cases in the history books of medicine of women whose third or even fourth breast was sufficiently well developed to feed an infant and during the Dark Ages these poor unfortunates were burnt at the stake as witches, as it was conventional wisdom in those days that these supernumerary breasts were used to feed the witches' familiar spirits. Much more common, however, are supernumerary nipples, which may often pass unremarked as skin blemishes or 'warts'.

Structure of the breast

The breast tissue itself is composed of variable proportions of secreting, glandular tissue and fatty (adipose) tissue. The secreting glandular tissue is divided up into 15 to 20 lobes, each lobe containing many hundreds of lobules (Figure 1). These are all connected together by small ducts (ductules) which further join together close to the nipple to produce the major lactiferous ducts which dilate out into the lactiferous sinuses, narrowing again as they pass through the nipple to form the seven or so duct openings.

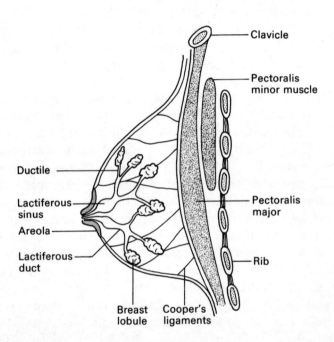

Fig. 1. Cross-section of breast

The breast tissue itself is enveloped in two layers of fibrous tissue, the deep layer overlying the muscle and the very thin superficial layer beneath the skin (see Figure 2). Joining these two layers are the fine fibrous ligaments, named after Sir Astley Cooper, which support the breast against the chest. After multiple pregnancies and lactation, or as a result of increasing obesity and age, Cooper's ligaments become stretched and the breast evolves from its virginal firmness to pendulous old age. In contrast, the earliest sign of some cancers may be the infiltration and shrinkage of Cooper's ligaments by the tumour, resulting in dimpling or puckering of the skin. A small extension of the breast tissue proper commonly wraps round the outer border of the pectoralis major muscle (see below) at the upper outer margin of the breast to form the so-called 'axillary tail', which is a not uncommon site for cancers.

Muscles

The principal muslces that are related to the breast are the pectoralis major, the pectoralis minor, the serratus anterior, and the latissimus dorsi (see Figure 2). The pectoralis major lies immediately under the breast covered in its thick sheet of fibrous tissue. It arises from the inner half of the collar-bone, the sternum (breast bone), and the sixth and seventh ribs at the front. It is a bulky triangular muscle which from this wide origin is inserted into a relatively narrow area on a rounded projection of the bone in the upper arm, the humerus. The muscle is responsible for the contour of the chest wall and forms the front (anterior) border of the axilla (armpit). The muscle is one of those groups responsible for pulling the arm in towards the chest. Deep to the pectoralis major is the pectoralis minor, a small muscle which arises from the third, fourth, and fifth ribs and is inserted into the front of the shoulder blade (scapula). The muscle has no very important action but is partly responsible for stabilizing the shoulder girdle. In the base of the armpit are two major muscles: the serratus anterior, which arises from the ribs at the side of the chest and is inserted into the scapula, and the large latissimus dorsi muscle which has a broad origin from the backbone and is inserted in the humerus forming the boundary at the back of the axilla. Damage to the nerve supply of these last two muscles during radical surgery to the breast can result in instability and winging of the shoulder blades.

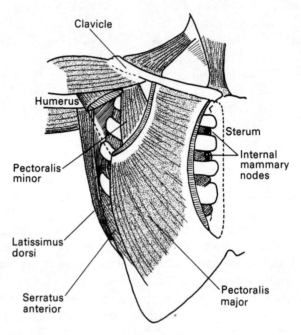

Fig. 2. The muscles in the chest wall

Blood supply

The blood supply to the breast comes from two major sources. First, there are branches running down the chest wall on the inner surface of the armpit from the axillary artery which runs across the apex of the armpit and supplies the outer half of the breast. The inner half of the breast is predominantly supplied by two or three small arteries that pass through the spaces between the second, third, and fourth ribs. These arteries arise from the internal mammary artery, which is itself a relatively minor branch of the major vessels coming off the aorta at the root of the neck. The venous drainage of the breast follows its arterial supply.

18

Structure and function of the breast

Lymph system

Lymph is the accumulation of tissue fluids between the cells of any organ. It is usually free of red blood cells except in cases of injury, but may be rich in protein and white blood cells. Lymph is collected in microscopic, thin-walled vessels forming the lymphatic drainage of the organ. In the breast the lymph flows centrifugally away from the nipple via a plexus of channels under the areolus, following the blood vessels towards the lymph glands (nodes) in the armpit and deep in the spaces between the ribs. Lymph from the outer quadrants of the breast flows into the axillary lymph nodes and then in stages through the various sub-groups of lymph nodes in the armpit, joining the lymphatic nodes in the neck via communication at the apex of the armpit between the collar-bone and the first rib. Lymph from the central quadrants of the breast, that is the inner half, flows towards the sternum and then through the spaces between the ribs to be drained via the lymph nodes that are intimately related to the internal mammary artery.

The lymph node

The lymph node is a structure approximately the shape and size of a kidney bean although varying in weight as a result of normal reactivity or involvement in disease processes. The lymph enters the node through multiple tiny channels and usually leaves the node through a single channel at the concave border. The node itself is composed predominantly of two cell types, lymphocytes (white blood cells) and histiocytes (macrophages) which are both known to be involved in various immune mechanisms. This tiny organ is now recognized to be biologically very active, with a role in the filtration of bacteria and toxic products and with involvement also in the various mechanisms of humoral and cellular immunity that are beyond the scope of this short book. However, there is still considerable controversy raging over whether or not

19

the lymphatic tissue has an important biological role in controlling cancer cells. Does the structure act as a filter, preventing the cancer cells from spreading in the flowing lymph beyond this anatomical position, or, alternatively, do the lymphocytes and histiocytes within the organ have an active role in the destruction of the cancer cell?

Structures removed at surgery

It is convenient at this point to mention briefly the structures which are removed in the various operations in the management of breast cancer.

1. *The simple or total mastectomy* removes all the breast tissue including the axillary tail and including an ellipse of skin containing the nipple and the areola. It is now conventional to take small samples of few of the lowermost axillary lymph nodes that are conveniently to hand at the termination of this procedure. The elliptical skin incision is then closed as a transverse line.

2. *The modified radical mastectomy* again removes all the breast tissue, but in addition removes the pectoralis minor muscle, thus gaining ease of access to the armpit so that all its contents, which include the lymph nodes within a pad of fat, may be cleaned out. After the operation the retention of the pectoralis major, and the transverse linear scar, make it impossible to distinguish from the simple mastectomy.

3. *The classical or Halsted radical mastectomy* removes the pectoralis major and pectoralis minor muscles and all the axillary lymphatic tissue. Postoperatively there is a concavity beneath the collar-bone where the ribs, which are normally covered by the pectoralis muscles, can be seen.

4. *The extended or super-radical mastectomy* includes all the tissue that would be removed at the Halsted mastectomy, but in addition a flap is lifted from the chest wall just alongside the sternum to allow the clearance of the lymphatic tissue which runs adjacent to the internal mammary artery.

20

Structure and function of the breast

Function of the breast

Although all males have some rudimentary mammary tissue, the development of the breast at adolescence can be considered the most important secondary sexual characteristic in females. That aside, the primary function of the breast is as an organ of lactation. To achieve this function the breast tissue is highly sensitive to changes in the levels of a large variety of naturally occurring hormones.

At adolescence, largely under the influence of the developing ovaries, the breast tissue enlarges, the milk ducts enlarge, and the branching system of ductules increases in size and number terminating in the glandular tissue of the lobules that are primed for further development at the time of pregnancy. Throughout the menstrual cycle the glandular tissue of the breast undergoes monthly changes, so that many women will notice that their breasts feel engorged, tender, and nodular in the week just before a period. Enormous proliferation of the lobular structure occurs in the early months of pregnancy and a variety of complex changes occur just before the baby is born in preparation for lactation. As long as the baby is suckling the endocrine system is stimulated to continue to produce milk and once suckling ceases, or as a result of the artificial termination of lactation by giving hormone tablets, involution occurs whereby the lobules decrease in size and number and the breast tissue as a whole shrinks.

After the menopause most of the glandular structures within the breast atrophy and are replaced by fatty tissue. However, many women retain considerable amounts of duct and glandular tissue within the breasts into old age. It has to be recognized, therefore, that the mammary tissue is constantly changing as a result of the normal aging process or as a result of the natural physiological alterations during the menstrual cycle, pregnancy, and lactation. These changes are activated and modulated by circulating hormones arising from the pituitary gland at the base of the brain, the ovaries, the adrenal glands sitting at the upper pole of the kidneys, and possibly hormones arising from the thyroid gland.

There are essentially two types of hormones — large molecules called proteins which account for the secretions of the pituitary gland and small molecules of a particular biochemical configuration referred to as steroid hormones and which arise from the ovaries and the adrenal glands. There are three different cell types within the breast tissue which are sensitive to various hormones. These are the cells lining the ducts, the glandular cells within the lobules, and the so-called myoepithelial cells with the capacity to contract, which are found as the network wrapped around the lobules having a role in the expression of milk from the gland into the duct collecting system.

The hormones act on the cells via two types of receptor mechanisms (see Figure 3). The protein hormones, which are too large to pass through the cell membrane, bind to receptors on the surface of the cell and this linkage induces enzyme activity, leading to the synthesis of a second messenger in the cell itself, triggering off a complex set of reactions within the nucleus with the end-result of protein synthesis.

The steroid hormones diffuse across the cell membrane and bind to specific high-affinity receptor proteins within the cell. The receptor–steroid complex is then translocated to the nucleus of the cell, again triggering off a complex series of reactions leading to the synthesis of RNA, which ultimately contributes to the manufacture of protein, and DNA, which leads to replication of genetic material of the cell itself and hence cell multiplication. The RNA so induced acts as a template for the manufacture of proteins, which include the specific milk proteins produced by the lobular cells, including casein and lactalbumin. In addition, the protein synthesis also leads to a replenishment of the steroid receptors themselves. The receptor for oestradiol, the major hormone secreted by the ovaries, is the one that has been most widely studied in relation to cancer of the breast and its relevance is discussed in more detail later on in this book.

Structure and function of the breast

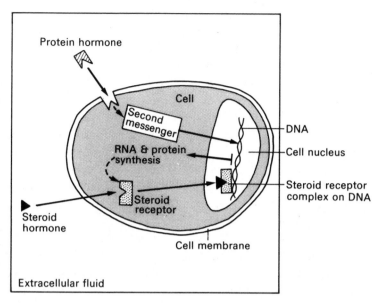

Fig. 3. Mechanisms of action of hormones upon cells

Endocrine influence on the development of the breasts at puberty, pregnancy, and the menopause

When a young girl reaches approximately 40 kg in weight, puberty is initiated. The pituitary starts to produce follicle stimulating hormone (FSH) and luteinizing hormone (LH). As a result of this, follicles are induced within the ovaries and as they mature they produce oestrogens, the most important of which is 17-beta-oestradiol. Under the influence of these oestrogens, mammary growth occurs: rudimentary ducts enlarge and branch to produce mature glandular tissue. Once the young girl starts ovulating a yellow patch replaces the ovarian follicle as each ovum is shed midway during the menstrual cycle. This structure is known as the corpus luteum, and is responsible for producing the steroid hormone progesterone. Progesterone has a secondary function in the maturation of the glandular tissues within the breast. Once the breast is fully developed, cyclical changes occur with each ovulation due to varying levels of the hormone prolactin arising from the pituitary and the ovarian hormones, oestradiol and progesterone. It is quite normal for women to be aware of these cyclical changes in the breast and many young girls are sufficiently alarmed to seek medical advice. It is sometimes difficult to judge when these natural physiological changes can be considered as abnormal, as there is no doubt that the benign mammary disease known as fibroadenosis, or fibrocystic disease, is a direct result of abnormal responses within the duct and glandular system of the breast to varying levels of pituitary and ovarian hormones.

During pregnancy the placenta is a rich source for the synthesis of hormones. Prolactin and growth hormone from the pituitary increase production and the placental hormone also influences the development of the glandular tissue within the breast. The ducts and lobules proliferate enormously in size and number and the breast is fully primed for the production of milk but is inhibited as a result of the placental hormone gonadotrophin. Following delivery of the baby and the placenta, this inhibition is removed and suckling further stimulates the pituitary not only to produce the protein hormones necessary for the synthesis of milk, but also to secrete the hormone oxytocin which acts on the myeoepithelial cells, allowing the glandular structures to empty of milk. Prolactin continues to stimulate the glandular cells to synthesize the milk proteins and oxytocin promotes the emptying of the glands so that they do not become engorged. Following the cessation of suckling, or alternatively by the administration of pharmacological doses of oestrogens, inhibition of the pituitary hormone secretion occurs and lactation ceases.

Later in life, following the menopause when ovarian function rapidly ceases, the fall in the level of circulating oestrogens and progesterones leads to involution and atrophy of glandular tissue in most cases and the breast is replaced by fat.

24

4

Benign and malignant changes and their symptoms

Introduction

It is probably appropriate at this point in the book to provide a glossary of terms that will facilitate the understanding of the rest of the text and in addition to explain just what the terms 'pathology' and 'cancer' mean.

Pathology is the study of disease processes. There is still considerable confusion amongst the lay public, the ancillary medical professions, and amongst doctors themselves as to the precise meaning of terms that are commonly used in relation to diseases of the breast. For example, such simple words as tumour, lesion, benign, and malignant are commonly tossed around by doctors in such a way as to confuse themselves, let alone their patients.

The word 'lesion' can be used in the manner of the caterpillar in Alice in Wonderland, to mean anything the doctor chooses it to mean. It is really a portmanteau word to refer to *any* disease process. The word 'tumour' is often used as a synonym for cancer, but this is totally inappropriate as the precise meaning of the word is swelling – which, pedantically speaking, can refer to diseases produced by inflammation, injury, or degeneration of tissues. Nevertheless, when the word tumour is preceded by the terms either benign or malignant, then we are usually referring to disease processes resulting from an abnormal growth of a group of cells within the body.

Benign tumours, as the word would suggest, are completely innocent, do not spread outside the organ of origin, and rarely lead to the death of the patient, although on occasions they may cause ugly deformity or damage to surrounding

25

tissues by pressure alone. Benign tumours are described by adding the suffix -oma to the name of the tissue from which it originates. The tissues of origin could be connective tissues, such as fat or fibrous material, or glandular tissue. An example of a benign connective tissue tumour would be a lipoma, arising from fat. These are very common and occasionally can occur in relation to the breast. The benign tumours arising from glandular tissues are described as adenomas and the one most commonly found in the breast, particularly in young girls, is referred to as a fibroadenoma, indicating that as well as glandular structures fibrous connective tissue is commonly seen as well.

The malignant tumours are the cancers. These are defined as abnormally growing cells which have the capacity for invasion of tissues within the local vicinity and dissemination via the lymphatic channels or the bloodstream. Cancers can either be primary or secondary: the primary cancer being the tumour at the site of origin and the secondary cancers, or metastases, the foci of malignant cells arrested in such organs as the liver or lung as a result of spread via the blood or lymphatic tissues.

Cancers of connective tissues are indicated by the suffix 'sarcoma', thus, for example, a malignant tumour of fibrous tissue is known as fibrosarcoma. These are, rarely, found within the breast, possibly as a result of malignant change within the pre-existing fibroadenoma. Cancers of epithelial or glandular tissue are indicated by the suffix 'carcinoma' and therefore the commonest cancer arising from the cells lining the ducts of breast tissue is known as the adenocarcinoma. Doctors commonly use euphemistic terms to discuss breast cancer in front of patients; the terms neoplasm (strictly speaking new growth) or mitotic lesion (indicating rapidly dividing cells) are the commonest euphemisms applied in this context.

Benign and malignant changes and their symptoms

Benign tumours of the breast

The commonest benign tumours of the breast are listed in Table 2. As already mentioned, young girls in the age group 15–25 may consult their doctor about a well-defined lump that feels like marble within the breast tissue, which on pathological examination is nearly always found to be a fibroadenoma. They rarely grow to a large size and should on all occasions be removed, first to exclude the remote possibility that they are cancers, and secondly because of the very slight worry that if neglected a small percentage will undergo malignant transformation to a sarcoma.

Table 2. *Benign breast disease*

Benign neoplasia	Fibroadenoma
	Lipoma
	Duct papilloma
	Skin lesions
Dysplasia	Fibrocystic disease
	Fibroadenosis
	('Chronic mastitis')
	Solitary cysts
Inflammatory disease	Puerperal abscess
	Periductal ('plasma cell') mastitis
	Tuberculosis
Trauma	Haematoma
	Fat necrosis
Developmental	Supernumerary breast
	Absent breast
	Asymmetrical development

'Duct papillomas' are little warty growths that occur within the lactiferous ducts. The first symptom is a bloody or yellow discharge from the nipple. They can occur at all ages and should usually be removed, partly because of their nuisance value and partly because on rare occasions they may have malignant potential.

Lipomas of the breast have already been mentioned, but it is worth noting that the breasts, like the rest of the body, are covered in skin and have the same risk of developing the common skin tumours, such as sebaceous cysts. Developmental abnormalities, as mentioned in Chapter 2, may lead to the appearance of supernumerary breasts or nipples, but it is not uncommon for young pre-pubertal girls to be sent to the clinic by panicky mothers because of what is thought to be a tumour in the area under the nipple. Strong reassurance is all that is needed in these cases because it is not uncommon for the developing breast disc to appear in an asymmetrical fashion. On no account should surgical interference be considered in these young girls of the age of 11–13 as this would inevitably lead to the absence or deformed development of the breast at puberty.

The most difficult subgroup of benign tumours within the breast as far as descriptive purposes are concerned are referred to in general terms as the mammary dysplasias. As explained in the section on the physiology of the breast in Chapter 2, there are problems in deciding when the normal physiological changes in the breast become established pathological abnormalities. Certainly, in their extreme form, lumpy areas that have been removed from the breast and examined under the microscope may show excessive proliferation of fibrous tissue and glandular tissue, with the formation of multiple small cysts. This type of disease has generated a profusion of pathological descriptive terms, such as fibroadenosis or fibrocystic disease, and used to be known as chronic mastitis. These extreme physiological/pathological changes of the mammary dysplasias may commonly be associated with pain in the breast which is described by doctors as either mastalgia or mastodynia.

On occasions these benign dysplastic changes may be dominated by a proliferation of the epithelial cells lining the milk ducts. This is known as epithelial hyperplasia and at its most extreme form is considered to be the only truly premalignant condition of the breast glandular structure.

One of the commonest benign tumours (using tumour to

mean swelling in this instance) is the solitary cyst. It is commonly found amongst women in the 35–55 age group. The cyst may be so tense as to fool the doctor into thinking that he is dealing with a solid mass, but the condition can be diagnosed and treated with confidence by simple needle aspiration of the contents. The cause of this common condition remains unknown.

Inflammation of the breast (mastitis) is relatively common and the best-recognized diseases are the acute bacterial infections within the duct system that may be associated with the late stages of pregnancy and the early stage of lactation. Unless the process is aborted very early on by inhibiting lactation and prescribing antibiotics, an abscess may eventually develop. Less common and less well recognized is the condition known as plasma cell mastitis (periductal mastitis) which is not of bacterial origin but is thought to be related to the leakage of protein-containing material from the duct system into the periductal tissue, setting up a chemical inflammation leading to the accumulation of inflammatory cells, amongst which the plasma cell (the antibody-producing cell) predominates.

Chronic inflammation of the breast is relatively rare, but may result from the inappropriate continued use of antibiotics in a young woman who has developed a breast abscess in the puerperium. I refer to this condition as an antibioma and the condition is best treated by withdrawing the antibiotics and applying heat to the breast to try and promote liquefication of the abscess. Infection of the breast with tubercle bacilli is extremely rare in developed countries. It may occur in the Indian sub-continent and among immigrant populations.

Finally, injury to the breast may produce lumps such as a haematoma, which is really a collection of blood within the breast tissue, and, rarely, severe injury may cause necrosis (cellular death) of the fat and this is supposed to produce a lump that can mimic a cancer. I personally am sceptical as to the clinical relevance of this pathological entity. However,

29

it is appropriate to conclude this section by emphasizing that women anxious about the lumps in their breasts will attempt to rationalize them away on the basis of pre-existing damage. The breasts are appendages which commonly get in the way of a working woman and are therefore commonly subjected to knocks and bumps. I always teach my students to ignore a history of such injury and treat each lump in the breast as a cancer until proved otherwise.

Malignant tumours of the breast (see Table 3)

For the purpose of this discussion it is appropriate first to dispose of two extremely rare varieties of breast cancer. First, the secondary deposit, or metastasis, arising from a cancer elsewhere in the body, and secondly, the malignant tumours of connective tissue origin which are termed sarcomata. Putting those curiosities on one side, we can then concentrate on the cancers arising from the cells lining the milk ducts or constituting the lobule of the glandular portion of the milk-producing apparatus.

Table 3. *Primary malignant breast disease*†

Duct origin	Pre-invasive	Intraduct cancer
	Invasive	Invasive duct cancer 'scirrhous cancer'
		Rare sub-types: Tubular Mucinous Medullary
Lobule origin	Pre-invasive	Lobular carcinoma *in situ*
	Invasive	Lobular invasive carcinoma
Connective tissue origin		Sarcoma (rare)

† Secondary tumours of the breast are rare

Pathologists generally recognize a pre-invasive variety of each type of cancer in which the malignant cells are confined entirely within the ducts or lobules in which they originated with no evidence of invasion into the surrounding tissue: this is described as an intraduct cancer, or lobular carcinoma *in situ*. Untreated there is good evidence that a high proportion of such cases will progress to frankly invasive cancer, but if excised at this stage in its evolution the outlook for the woman is excellent.

Lobular invasive cancers are relatively uncommon, perhaps accounting for 8 per cent of all cancers, and are frequently associated with multi-centred invasive or pre-invasive changes within the same breast or the opposite breast, but otherwise behave in a similar fashion to the invasive duct adenocarcinoma. This latter group probably accounts for 90 per cent of all malignant tumours arising within the breast so I will describe its symptoms and appearance, both on simple observation and under the microscope, and its mode of spread.

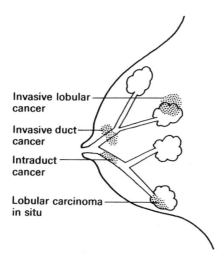

Invasive lobular cancer

Invasive duct cancer

Intraduct cancer

Lobular carcinoma in situ

Fig. 4. Types of breast cancer

Symptoms of invasive duct cancer

The earliest detectable change produced by an invasive duct cancer is of a hard, somewhat ill-defined *lump* occurring within the breast. As the tumour invades locally it infiltrates along the ligaments of Astley Cooper (see Figure 1), pulling in the overlying skin to produce a characteristic *dimple*. It may also invade along the lactiferous ducts, causing these to shrink and thus *invert the nipple*. Further local infiltration will ultimately lead to fixation or even ulceration of the skin overlying the tumour and as the cancer invades deeply, the mass may eventually become fixed to the underlying muscles or even to the structures of the chest wall. Widespread infiltration within the breast may produce oedema (excess fluid) of the overlying skin, causing it to thicken, with many small dimples at the site of insertion of Cooper's ligaments, giving the appearance of orange skin (*peau d'orange*), which is a clinical sign of grave significance. Spread of the cancer into the axillary lymph nodes leads to the appearance of large hard lumps within the armpit and occasionally these local deposits themselves can infiltrate and ulcerate the skin.

These gross clinical changes have been used as a crude method of assessing outlook, being referred to as the clinical stages of the disease. The earliest stages are presented merely by a palpable lump with no fixation to the deep structures or the overlying skin, and no clinically apparent axillary lymph node involvement. Locally advanced stages are indicated by fixation or ulceration of the skin and fixation of the tumour to the underlying structures, with or without the gross involvement of axillary lymph nodes. There is no doubt that the smaller and less advanced the tumour is at the time of diagnosis, the better the survival prospects for the patient irrespective of treatment.

The appearance of the cancer in a specimen of the tissue removed at mastectomy is very characteristic. In the majority of cases the tumour has a grey, granular, or gritty cut surface, with radiating spicules often giving the characteristic crab-like appearance from which cancer earns its name. Less commonly the tumour is well circumscribed and clearly defined, under which circumstances it can masquerade as a benign tumour.

Microscopic appearance of breast cancer

The microscopic, or histological, appearance of breast cancer is very characteristic and seldom causes any diagnostic problem. The cancer cells appear as irregular columns or pockets of abnormal-looking cells scattered throughout a background of fibrous connective tissue. The dense fibrous tissue accounts for the hard feel of the cancer and also accounts for the descriptive term 'scirrhous' (GK *skirros* = hard) which is often applied to the commonest types of breast malignancy.

Cancer cells can demonstrate a whole spectrum of differentiation. At one extreme recognizable ducts and tubules are formed by the malignant cells that may retain sufficient characteristics of the structure of origin as to secrete mucus. These rare varieties of breast cancer, known as tubular and mucinous cancers, carry an excellent outlook. At the other extreme, the cells are so de-differentiated as to be unrecognizable as arising from the duct epithelium. These cancers are described as 'anaplastic' and carry the worst outlook. The degree of differentiation of the cancer seen under the microscope is referred to as the *grade* of malignancy and in the hands of an expert pathologist can give a fairly reliable guide to outlook for the patient independent of the clinical stage of the disease. In addition to the cancer cells and the fibrous framework, it is commonplace to see other varieties of cells, such as lymphocytes and histiocytes, which are thought by some to reflect the body's natural reaction to the presence of the cancer cells (An extreme variety of this type of cancer, where lymphocytes predominate, is known as medullary carcinoma of the breast.) At one time it was thought that the degree of infiltration by host immune cells was another reliable, independent guide to outlook. Although a very attractive hypothesis, recent evidence from many large studies has failed to corroborate the suggestion.

Breast cancer is truly a heterogeneous collection of diseases behaving in an unpredictable manner with extreme clinical variability. Conventional clinical staging and histological grading of the cancer go only a small way towards the accurate prediction of prognosis for the individual patient. Exciting new work aimed at interpreting the biological activity and growth potential of individual cancers is under way, but a full description of these new techniques is outside the scope of this volume.

Modes of spread of breast cancer

The local invasion of breast cancer by direct infiltration has already been described, but the lethal propensity of the disease results from its capacity to shed single or clumps of cells, which can develop into cancers at distant sites in the body. The modes of spread are predominantly along the lymphatic channels and the bloodstream. These two systems, once thought to be entirely independent of one another, are now recognized to be intimately related and communications between the lymphatics and veins would suggest that either portal of entry into the patient's system could allow the establishment of secondary or metastatic deposits anywhere within the body. Undoubtedly the commonest site for early secondary involvement is the regional lymph nodes. From involvement of one lymph node it is likely that cells can escape via the exit lymphatic channels into a more distant group of lymph nodes, eventually spreading up the axilla and into the base of the neck. Alternatively, tumours in the inner quadrants of the breast can spread through the internal mammary chain of lymphatic tissue and perhaps from there into the chest cavity itself, leading to the involvement of tissue of the lungs or around the heart, which may produce the complications of fluid in the chest or cavities around the heart. Histological evidence of invasion of the regional lymph nodes is regarded as a very grave sign and it is now widely accepted that extensive involvement of the nodes in the axilla is symptomatic that the disease is already widespread via the bloodstream to the vital organs. External palpation of the axilla can on occasions be very misleading as the enlarged lymph nodes that are felt may not in fact contain cancer, but may be exhibiting so-called 'reactive hyperplasia', where the lymph node is swollen by cells of the immune system (lymphocytes and histiocytes); this again has been suggested as part of the putative natural resistance to the spread of cancer.

The most important mode of spread determining the final outcome of treatment is via the bloodstream, probably as a result of direct invasion into the veins draining the breast. Not all cells shed from the cancer into the blood are necessarily viable or clonogenic (that is having the capacity to develop into metastatic deposits). Those viable cancer cells that do escape may lodge in the bone, the liver, the lungs, or the brain, thus contributing to the patient's death in a number of ways (e.g. bone marrow failure, liver failure, or respiratory failure). So protean are the manifestations of metastatic breast cancer that the patient could be referred to any number of specialists depending on the dominant site of secondary disease. Therefore, all doctors need to be on the alert that patients presenting with such diverse symptoms as jaundice or spontaneous fractures of the long bones may in fact be suffering from the same primary disease, namely invasive duct cancer of the breast.

5

Screening and self-examination

A breast cancer has the potential to spread and form secondary growths almost from the date of its inception. Thus, a mutant cell arising from the lactiferous ducts, having undergone only two divisions, could in theory release into the circulation one of the new line of malignant cells capable of cloning, which, should it lodge within a vital organ, would be the ultimate cause of the woman's death. Assuming that breast cancer can demonstrate a broad spectrum of such behaviour, as described in the previous chapter, then the tumour could disseminate at any interval in its growth from the size of, say, 40 micrometres (tenth of a pinhead) in diameter until after it has assumed a clinically detectable lump of more than 2 centimetres.

However, it would seem reasonable to hope that by screening large populations of women within the breast cancer age group by a combination of mammography and clinical examination it would be possible to pick up subclinical tumours which have not yet had the opportunity to metastasize. To test this hypothesis, a very important study was established by the Health Insurance Plan in New York just over ten years ago. The women were divided randomly into two groups of 31 000 each: one group received annual screening by mammography and the other group was used as a control population and allowed to come forward with their breast cancers found by self-detection. As might have been predicted, smaller cancers with a lower incidence of involvement of lymph nodes were picked up amongst the screened population, with an ultimate reduction in mortality rates from breast cancer after seven years of follow-up. Unfortunately, the benefit appeared to apply only to the women over the age of 50,

Screening and self-examination

and even amongst the screened population cancers which appeared to be of the more aggressive type developed between the fixed screening intervals, reducing, though by no means abolishing, the benefit of the annual screen that was demonstrated by the whole of the test population. From this experiment there can be little doubt that screening can save lives, but a fierce controversy is still raging as to the cost–benefit ratio of such exercises.

For the intelligent layman it seems inconceivable that screening and early detection can do anything but good, but unfortunately many serious reservations exist. First of all, even if a screening programme exists for well women, a significant proportion of those invited will not attend either for fear that something *might* be found, or, alternatively, because they cannot be bothered with the inconvenience involved. At the same time it is noticeable that amongst the population of women who do accept the invitation for screening, there is a higher-than-expected incidence of those with symptoms who are merely using the screening clinic as an opportunity to come forward with their breast lump that had in any case been bothering them in the preceding interval. Furthermore, a negative finding at the first examination may create a false sense of security and once a screening programme has been established it is necessary that women should be invited back at regular intervals for the rest of their lives for follow-up examinations, although it is by no means sure what the optimum interval should be between screening examinations. An annual screen appears to be the convention in America, but this has no more scientific validity than any other interval of time, being based on the revolutions of the earth around the sun rather than any recognized biological property of breast cancer cells!

Inevitably, screening programmes will generate an increased biopsy rate, as many women with lumpy breasts due to benign disorders will be referred to the surgeon for minor operative procedures. Even the smallest breast operation causes great psychological stress, and as with a very large number of any type of operation, there might be a small percentage of surgical and anaesthetic mishaps.

Next we have to consider the risk of low doses of ionizing radiation affecting the breast. There is no doubt that radiation exposure can cause breast cancer, as discussed on page 13. There is no agreed safe dose of radiation, so it must be recognized that there is a very small risk of inducing cancers by repeating mammograms at intervals, perhaps extending over 30 years. I do not feel that these risks should be exaggerated, and with new techniques delivering a very low dose of radiation (less than 1 rad) for a complete set of mammograms, and providing the mammograms are not repeated more often than once a year, many experts feel that the risks are being reduced to a safe minimum.

Another nagging anxiety about the screening programmes is the number of abnormalities of marginal significance that are now being detected. The histological diagnosis of cancer is not always cut and dried; many small mammographic changes on biopsy demonstrate minimal changes on the borderline between epithelial hyperplasia, intraduct cancer, and minimal invasive cancer. Often the pathologist and the surgeon are in doubt as to what should be the definitive management of such cases and it is likely, therefore, that in any large-scale screening programme a number of mastectomies will be carried out because abnormalities which if left alone would not progress to truly invasive cancer have been detected. With all the above reservations in mind, the Department of Health in the United Kingdom has very wisely set up a pilot screening programme in three different regions in the country to try to confirm the experience of the New York Health Insurance Plan Study.

Cost-effectiveness of screening

When calculating the cost-effectiveness of screening programmes we have to estimate the cost of each life saved as a result of the programme rather than the cost of each cancer detected. The latter is easy to estimate: the total cost of the screening programme, which includes, of course, the diagnostic equipment and the salaries of the professional groups involved, is divided up by the number of cancers found. Unfortunately, all cancers found in a screening programme are not curable, so to estimate the cost of each life saved it is necessary to divide the total cost of the programme by the number of curable cancers detected which are in excess of the number of curable cancers which might have been self-detected. Such estimates are extremely difficult to calculate and depend on all sorts of unverifiable assumptions. However, whichever way the calculations are arrived at, the cost of each additional life saved from a screening programme is quite enormous and probably in the region of £30–40 000 ($60–80 000). Many would argue that the value of life of a woman bringing up young children is far greater than £40 000 and, to quote the proverb: 'A woman of worth is valued higher than rubies'. Unfortunately, we cannot get away from the hard fact that at a time of economic recession and cutbacks in expenditure within the health services, many countries at the present cannot afford a national screening programme. For that reason alone we need to look for more effective ways of utilizing limited resources and also perhaps to define a particular high-risk population who would benefit from screening to a much greater extent than the general population of women in the 30–70 age group. Much current research is directed at this question and at the time of writing most experts would agree that childless women over the age of 30 with a family history of breast cancer might benefit from regular screening examinations.

Self-examination

A recent survey in the Cardiff Breast Clinic demonstrated that about 70 per cent of women with lumps in their breast had intentionally delayed reporting their symptoms to the family doctor. This delay varied from a few months to several years. In the vast majority of cases it was not ignorance that fostered the delay but more likely fear of having the diagnosis of cancer confirmed and a wish to delay or deny the inevitable. Most of this fear could be allayed by an intensive programme of public education that would encourage women to attend by pointing out that less than one in four of lumps in the breast turns out to be cancer. Many women live in dread when all they have is a simple cyst that could be diagnosed and treated by needle aspiration.

At the same time, if we accept that the earlier the presentation the less likely it is that the disease will have disseminated, then regular self-examination and prompt self-referral by the patient might save an equivalent number of lives as a very costly national screening programme. In making such an apparently outrageous statement it has to be remembered that nearly half of the breast cancers that are seen in the clinics are at an incurable stage, with primary tumours often in excess of 5 centimetres in diameter. Surely these tumours must have been easily detectable by the woman for long periods of time before presentation. I feel it is the responsibility of all health professionals to encourage women to practise self-examination. It should also be the responsibility of departments of health to ensure that there are adequate numbers of breast clinics where women with symptoms can be seen without any delay.

A system of self-examination published by the Women's National Cancer Council is fully illustrated in Plate 1.

6

Diagnosis

The majority of women who go to their doctor with breast symptoms complain of lumps in the breast, pain in the breast, or nipple discharge. The lump they complain of may be a solitary discrete abnormality, or more diffuse, occupying one or more quadrants of either breast. A discrete lump may be associated with deformity of the breast or indrawing of the nipple. Pain in the breast is commonly a symptom of young women, cyclical in nature, and at its peak in the pre-menstrual week. Occasionally the pain may be complained of as a constant, localized ache. Nipple discharge may be clear or blood-stained, from a solitary duct from one nipple, or of a variety of hues arising from multiple ducts of both nipples. Flow-charts showing patterns of management based on symptoms are shown in Figures 5–7.

A woman with a lump in the breast may often complain of recent blow or injury, but this is rarely relevant to the

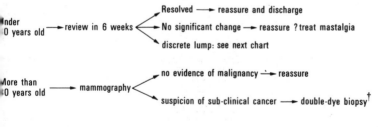

† Accurate technique used to localize an area thought from the mammogram to be suspicious, but impalpable, before biopsy

Fig. 5. Flow chart for diagnosis when a patient has no discrete breast lump, but complains of pain and/or nodularity

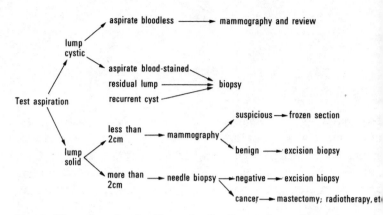

Fig. 6. Flow chart for the diagnosis of a discrete breast lump

diagnosis as it is commonly an attempt at rationalization, or, alternatively, the local injury may have drawn her attention to a previously existing abnormality.

In general terms, the statistical probabilities would suggest that a discrete lump in the breast of a woman over the age of 55 is likely to be a cancer and below the age of 30 is likely to be a benign tumour called a fibroadenoma (see Chapter 4). In the intervening years the most probable diagnosis is of a solitary cyst. Diffuse nodular or granular lumps may occur at almost any age and are usually associated with some form of benign abnormality or mammary dysplasia (such as fibroadenosis, chronic mastitis, or cystic hyperplasia). It cannot be emphasized strongly enough that these are broad statistical likelihoods and a precise histological or cytological diagnosis must be made for all discrete breast lumps.

Clinical examination

The first step towards arriving at a diagnosis is a full and careful clinical examination. It is inappropriate in a book of this nature to attempt a textbook coverage of how the doctor examines the breasts in detail, but a few general points are

42

Diagnosis

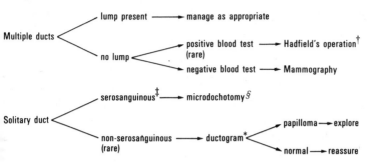

† *technique for removing a wedge of tissue, behind the nipple, containing terminal ducts*

‡ *mixture of blood and yellow serum*

§ *removal of a single lactiferous duct thought to contain a papilloma*

∗ *insertion of radio-opaque dye into lactiferous ducts for special X-rays*

Fig. 7. Flow chart for the diagnosis of nipple discharge

worth noting. First, the patient is observed from the front, sitting up with her hands first by her side and then raised above her head. In this way retraction of the nipple or asymmetry and dimpling of one of the breasts will be detected. Sadly, a large proportion of cancers can be diagnosed in this way before even the doctor lays hands upon the patient's breasts. Next, with the patient in a semi-recumbent position, both breasts are examined quadrant by quadrant with the flat of the hand. It is essential at this stage to decide whether a discrete lump does in fact exist or whether the woman has merely noted a change in texture, or the appearance of coarse nodular (lumpy) tissue within the breasts. This type of diffuse nodularity is a common feature of benign mammary dysplasia (Chapter 4) and predominantly affects the upper outer quadrants of the mammary glands. The doctor next carefully feels under both the woman's arms. If a cancer is suspected, a more intense search for disseminated disease is carried out in the depressions over the collarbone, by sounding the chest, and abdominal examination. If a nipple discharge is the initial complaint, then the woman should be asked to demonstrate the discharge by massaging the sub areolar area; the doctor makes a careful note of the colour and site of origin of the discharge. The serous or bloody discharge from a single duct almost invariably indicates a duct papilloma. Sometimes the presence of blood is not obvious to the naked eye and is revealed only by special tests.

Assuming a discrete lump can be felt, the next step is a test aspiration with a simple 20 ml syringe and venepuncture needle. Some cysts are so tense that they feel solid, so clinical examination in these cases could be misleading. Test aspiration is a simple and virtually painless procedure which can confirm the diagnosis and effectively cure the condition by one simple manoeuvre. The instant relief and reassurance the woman achieves as a result of this technique is very gratifying for the clinician. If the lump is in fact solid rather than liquid-filled and eventually turns out to be cancer there is no evidence that the outcome is prejudiced by needle puncture. The only caveat about this procedure is that failure of the lump to resolve fully, or the presence of a blood-stained aspirate, may indicate the presence of an intracystic cancer which should be dealt with by open biopsy, described at the end of this chapter.

Outpatient biopsy

If test aspiration demonstrates that the discrete lump is in fact solid, then ideally an attempt should be made there and then to get histological confirmation of the diagnosis. Perhaps the most important development in the diagnostic field in recent years has been the improvements in techniques for obtaining samples from suspicious lumps at the time of the first visit of the patient to the clinic. There are two methods that have to be considered. First, cutting-needle biopsy and secondly, aspiration cytology. Needle biopsy can easily be achieved from breast lumps greater than 1 centimetre in size

Diagnosis

After defining a discrete solid lump the skin is infiltrated with local anaesthetic, a small stab incision is made in the skin and the cutting needle is inserted into the centre of the lump (see Plate 2). In most cases an adequate core of material is obtained that can be subjected to routine histopathological examination. There are no false positives using this technique, but a negative result must be ignored and the lump dealt with by open biopsy (see p. 47).

Many centres in this country are experimenting with fine-needle aspiration suitable for the smallest of solid lumps. The material obtained is usually represented by a few clusters of cells. These are examined by special cytological stains and in expert hands this will be sufficient to establish a diagnosis of invasive cancer within a few minutes, whilst the patient is still at the clinic.

The advantages of the definitive diagnosis of cancer at the first visit of a woman to the clinic are enormous. A search for secondary growths can be established immediately, the surgeon can proceed with a full, frank discussion with the woman and her husband concerning the choice of surgery, the patient is spared the severe psychological trauma of being subjected to a general anaesthetic without knowing if she will awake with or without her breast.

Mammography

Modern mammographic (X-ray) techniques have achieved a very high degree of sophistication with a diagnostic accuracy for clinically detectable breast lumps in excess of 95 per cent and an accuracy rate in the order of 50 per cent for subclinical cancers. However, in spite of these remarkable achievements it still remains somewhat difficult to define the role of mammography outside the screening clinics. It should be stated quite dogmatically that irrespective of the mammographic diagnosis a discrete, palpable lump in the breast should be dealt with as described above. In the author's

45

view, therefore, mammography has no specific role to play in the management of a clinically obvious lump in the breast. Nonetheless, access to mammography remains vitally important to the specialist for a number of reasons.

1 If the breast has coarse nodular dysplasia it may be impossible to feel a relatively small carcinoma. Mammography is such cases would raise the index of suspicion.
2 In a woman with an obvious lump in the breast, mammography may demonstrate an impalpable carcinoma in the same breast or an unsuspected carcinoma in the other breast.
3 A woman who has already had a mastectomy for carcinoma of the breast stands a higher than normal chance of developing disease in her remaining breast. It is therefore reasonable to carry out mammography at regular intervals in the follow-up of a woman after mastectomy.

Other imaging techniques, such as thermography and ultrasonography, have proved to be somewhat disappointing in the diagnosis of breast cancer as they produce so many false-positive results. In the hands of a few enthusiasts they remain useful diagnostic tools, but it is unlikely that these alternative imaging techniques will contribute greatly to the management of carcinoma of the breast.

If clinical examination and mammography are negative, then all that needs to be done is to reassure the woman as strongly as possible. In particular those women with breast pain who are concerned that they have symptoms of cancer (which is in any case highly unlikely) need the firmest reassurance. In some cases, though, if there is a bad family history and other risk factors present, or if the mammographic findings show severe dysplastic changes which are thought to predispose to the development of malignancy, it would be reasonable to offer the woman annual re-examination.

Diagnosis

Open biopsy

In all cases where there are discrete lumps, suspicious nodularity, or suspicious mammographic findings, or where outpatient needle sampling has failed to demonstrate unequivocal cancer, the patient should be admitted to hospital as promptly as convenient for excisional biopsy under general anaesthesia. If clinical and radiographic findings are highly suspicious of cancer, then probably it is wise to forewarn the women and send the specimen for 'frozen section' which allows immediate reporting to confirm the cancer before proceeding to mastectomy. This conventional practice is becoming less and less common as outpatient diagnosis becomes more efficient. Those case which are clinically and mammographically benign are better managed by excision biopsy and careful histological examination rather than putting the woman through the agony of having to consent to mastectomy before the anaesthetic when there is only the smallest of chances that the lump is indeed a cancer. Adopting this policy, women need no longer worry that they will be rushed into a mastectomy before having had the opportunity to discuss with their husbands and the surgeon the operation or its alternatives.

7

The course of breast cancer

Before being in a position to interpret the effectiveness of treatment for carcinoma of the breast it is essential to know something about the natural history of the disease. By natural history we mean: 'how would the cancer progress without treatment?' This may appear a rather foolish question as it is widely assumed that untreated cancer of any kind must lead to the inevitable and rapid death of the patient in all cases. Although this may, indeed, be the case for cancer of the lung and cancer of the stomach, surprisingly, our knowledge of the natural history of breast cancer is imperfect, to say the least. The problems as far as breast cancer are concerned are threefold. First, it is unthinkable these days to withhold treatment from any woman with breast cancer and, therefore, we have to rely on information from the last century to estimate the natural history of the untreated disease. Secondly, we recognize that breast cancer can be a very slowly progressive disease, in spite of treatment, leading to the patient's death maybe 20 years after mastectomy. When we remember that the average age of onset is 55, it is not surprising, therefore, that a number of women will die of other causes, even though not 'cured' of their original cancer. Finally, we also recognize that the disease does not behave as a single entity but has an extraordinarily wide biological variation in behaviour, with some women dying of the disease with an almost undetectable primary tumour, whereas others may live for many years after having refused treatment in the first place.

Records of the nineteenth century

There are a number of quite reliable reports of the progression

48

of untreated breast cancer in the era before the standard use of mastectomy. In those days before Lister had introduced antisepsis into surgery and in the very early days of anaesthesia many doctors wisely refrained from referring their patients with breast tumours to the surgeon's knife. Gross, a famous surgeon in Philadelphia, published a beautifully clear report in 1880 of approximately 100 cases with breast tumours who received nothing other than constitutional 'support'. From this study, he described how skin infiltration appeared on average 14 months after a tumour was first detected. Ulceration of the skin occurred on average six months later and fixation of the tumour to the chest wall after a further two months. Invasion of the second breast was seen on average three years after the first lump appeared amongst those who survived long enough. The average time for the appearance of enlarged axillary nodes amongst those who presented with Stage I disease (see Table 5) was 15 months. Twenty-five per cent of these untreated cases developed distant metastases within one year, but for a similar percentage of cases distant metastases did not occur until after three years from initial presentation. This and many similar series of the same era described a 10 per cent ten-year survival without any treatment.

More recently a very interesting study was reported by Dr. Bloom of the Royal Marsden Hospital in London. He studied the records of 250 women who died of breast cancer in the Middlesex Hospital cancer ward between 1905 and 1933. Nearly all of these patients were admitted to the ward with either locally advanced or widely disseminated disease. He calculated the survival rates from the alleged onset of the symptoms until the patient's death in the cancer ward. He estimated that 18 per cent survived five years and 3.6 per cent ten years, with the average survival of the whole group being a little over three years.

There are several criticisms that can be levelled against all these studies so far quoted, which perhaps invalidate their use as a baseline against which to judge the curative effect of conventional therapy. There must have been an element of selection for withholding treatment even in the period before Lister, so that the majority of cases, with the exception of those who actively refused help, might have been judged to have a poor outlook to begin with. Secondly, all these cases represent women seeking medical attention at a time before public health education had warned the population of the sinister significance of breast lumps. It is likely, therefore, that many women were content to co-exist with their breast lumps until they died of old age or were knocked down by a hansom cab. So that, in effect, these historical reports refer to the natural history of large or locally advanced breast cancers rather than the natural history of the patient who presents with a 2-centimetre lump in modern times. Support for this viewpoint can be extracted from a statistical review of the Ontario Cancer Clinics published in 1965. Within this study of nearly 10 000 cases it was possible to pick out 50 women who presented with early breast cancer and refused treatment for a variety of reasons. This group apparently enjoyed a nearly 70 per cent five-year survival after the time of first symptom, a figure that does not compare unfavourably with many of the treated series in contemporary literature. It is not inconceivable, therefore, that in the broadest general terms breast cancers exhibit two behaviour patterns: one group that metastasizes very early on and must be judged incurable by any form of local treatment and a second group that is non-metastasizing, or at the worst does not start to metastasize until the lump has been obvious for a number of years, which might be curable by any form of surgery or radiotherapy.

If such is the case, when can a woman be judged to be cured from her breast cancer following mastectomy? Halsted initially felt that a three-year follow-up was adequate before pronouncing the woman cured, and although it is true that there is an accelerated death rate in the first three years after mastectomy, subsequent experience has demonstrated just how fallacious was this early pronouncement. Today it is conventional when describing the results of treatment to talk about ten-year survival rates, as if these in some way indicate the proportion of women cured of their disease, but unfortunately it is not as easy as that. A classical study by Dr. Brinkley and Dr. Haybittle followed up over 700 cases of breast cancer treated by radical mastectomy in the Cambridge area over a 25-year period. Making allowances for the fact that many women during this follow-up time would die of old age and incidental disease, they estimated that the excess risk of dying over an age-matched population as a result of the original breast cancer did not disappear until after 20 years had passed. This led some cynics to suggest that a woman has not been cured of her breast cancer until she has died of some other disease! From Brinkley and Haybittle's very careful analysis, it is reasonable to conclude that approximately 30 per cent of women presenting with 'early' carcinoma of the breast and subjected to mastectomy will have a normal expectation of life. Bearing in mind that little more than half of the cases of breast cancer that surgeons see fall within the 'early' stages of the disease, we are left with the rather depressing conclusion that overall only about 15 per cent of breast cancer cases referred to the clinics are 'cured' by conventional therapy. However, unlike cancer of the lung and cancer of the stomach, many of the women who may eventually be judged as incurable can be expected to live for a considerable number of years in comfort as a result of modern therapeutic strategy, which would at least allow them to see their children through school or be around to advise on the upbringing of their first grandchild.

To illustrate the extreme variability in the natural history of carcinoma of the breast I have chosen two cases. The first was a charming 90-year-old woman who first sought medical advice for a lump in the breast 30 years previously. On this occasion carcinoma was diagnosed and she was advised to have a radical mastectomy. She declined this advice and has remained hale and hearty until the present time. During all this period the original tumour grew at a slow but steady rate, and she also developed a second tumour in her other breast. She managed to outlive the surgeon who advocated mastectomy and, in addition, outlived three husbands. There was still no clinical or radiological evidence of distant dissemination when she eventually appeared in my clinic. It is unlikely that radical mastectomy 30 years ago would have improved on this outcome. Microscopic examination of a sample of the tumour removed by needle biopsy showed tubular carcinoma, a pathological sub-type of breast cancer which is known to carry an excellent prognosis. Other pathological sub-groups, such as mucinous or medullary carcinoma of the breast, are also known to possess a relatively good prognosis, but I have also come across other patients with unspecified invasive duct cancer who had refused treatment in the past and yet lived with slowly progressing local disease for upwards of 12 years without evidence of dissemination.

The other extreme is illustrated by a 45-year-old premenopausal woman who first complained to her family doctor of general discomfort and breathlessness on exertion. Clinically she appeared anaemic and was referred to the Haematology Department. Examination of the peripheral blood showed abnormal red and white blood cells indicative of malignant disease and aspiration of the bone marrow confirmed infiltration with malignant cells. The most careful clinical evaluation of the patient failed to reveal a primary malignancy. Eventually X-rays of the breast were requested and these demonstrated three minute foci of cancer (Plate 3). Open biopsy finally confirmed the diagnosis; she was treated initially by removal of her ovaries (see Chapter 7) and demonstrated a worth while and prolonged remission, but sadly died 18 months after her first visit to her doctor.

Within these two extreme ends of the spectrum fall the majority of cases; one can perhaps deduce from this that

Inspection — How to look

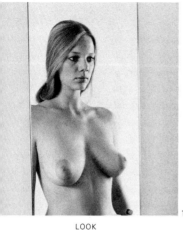

LOOK

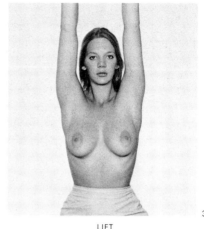

LIFT

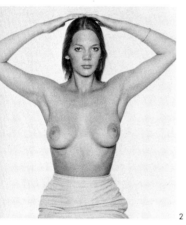

STRETCH

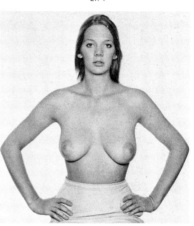

PRESS

Undress to the waist and sit or stand in front a mirror in a good light with your arms nfortably by your sides. If sitting, you may find referable to rest your hands lightly on your hips. k at your breasts carefully; In the first mination you should note the normal size and pe of each breast and the position of the les so that you will be aware of any changes t might develop. In subsequent examinations J should look for any inequality in the size or pe of your breasts. Pay special attention to any rations in the surface of the breast, such as a lling, skin puckering (dimple), rash, colouration or very prominent veins. Note ether either nipple is retracted (turned in). Now place the hands lightly on the top of the d and again look at the breasts carefully, ncentrating especially on the nipples. This

position will emphasise any difference in size or shape between the two breasts. Look particularly for any excessive upward or outward movement of either nipple.
3. Momentarily stretch the arms above the head. Again this will emphasise any difference between the two breasts.
4. Now place the hands firmly on your hips and, when you are comfortable, push inwards towards the hips. You should feel the muscles on the upper part of your chest beneath your breasts tighten when you do this. Look at the breasts carefully while you keep pressing. This movement will emphasise any puckering of the skin or any abnormal retraction of either nippple. Remember to look at the under surface of the breast during this part of the examination. It is often easier to stand up to do this properly.

ate 1   Breast self-examination leaflet produced by the Women's National Cancer Control Campaign (United Kingdom)

Palpation — How to feel

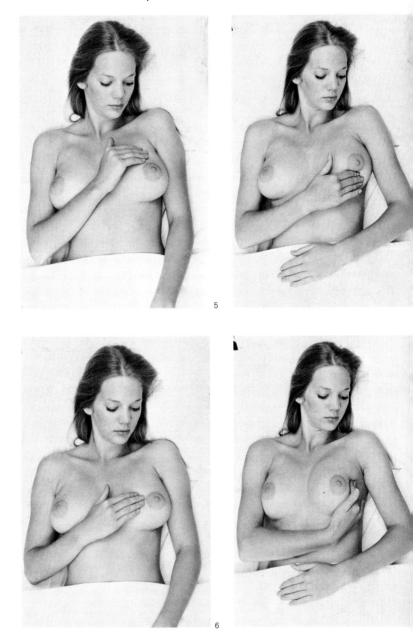

Plate 1 (cont.)   Breast self-examination

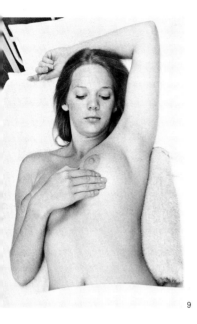

You have completed the INSPECTION part of the examination and it is now time to feel for any abnormal lumps in the breasts. Again it is important at the first examination to note the normal consistency of your breasts, so that you will be aware of any change in subsequent examinations. Many women who have not yet reached the change of life normally have rather lumpy breasts just before the period and in some this may persist throughout the whole month. This may cause uncertainty at first, but with each successive examination it should become easier to decide whether any unusual lump is present.

5. Lie down comfortably on a firm surface with your head on a pillow. Place a folded towel under the shoulder slightly raising the side that you are going to examine first. The left breast is felt with your right hand and vice versa. The first part of the examination is done with the arm by the side. Feel with the flat of the pads of the middle three fingers. The fingers should be kept straight but the hand flexible. Each time you feel, the breast tissue should be pressed towards the chest wall. Firm but gentle pressure should be used.

6. 7. 8. The examination starts just above the nipple and continues outward in a spiral fashion around the breast. EVERY PART of the breast must be felt so that two or three complete circles will need to be made depending on the size of the breast. Any unusual discrete lump or nodule should be noted.

9. It is not easy to examine the most outer part of the breast with the arm by the side. When you have completed the first series of circular movements place the arm comfortably above the head with the elbow bent. Repeat the examination of all the breast now, paying especial attention to the outer part which can now be felt with more certainty. Never rush palpation of the breasts which must be done slowly, gently, and thoroughly.

10. The final part of the examination is of the so-called tail of the breast which extends towards the armpit. This can only be examined properly with the arm above the head.

You have now completed palpation of one breast and this must be repeated for the other side.

Having completed self-examination of your breasts you will have decided whether they remain unchanged or whether any unusual feature has appeared. To remind you of these features, they are again listed overleaf.

9

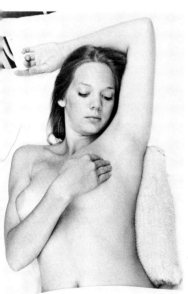

10

Plate 1 (cont.)   Breast self-examination

Warning Signs

ON INSPECTION

Unusual difference in size or shape of the breasts.

Alterations in the position of either nipple.

Retraction (turning in) of either nipple.

Puckering (dimple) of the skin surface.

Unusual rash on the breast or nipple.

Unusual prominence of the veins over either breast.

ON PALPATION

Unusual discrete lump or nodule in any part of either breast.

Routine Examinations

Try to make the examination of your breasts a monthly habit. Immediately following a period would be a suitable time, or on the first day of the month if you have had the menopause.

Remember

Many women will have symptoms similar to those listed above. It won't necessarily be cancer — a lump may be just a simple cyst.
Breast cancer can be treated very successfully when it is diagnosed in the early stages. The success rate is now approaching 80% for early cases.

Early Detection

Your doctor or Area Health Authority clinic will be able to help you if you have any difficulty in following these diagrams. Your Health Visitor or the staff at your Family Planning clinic can also advise you.

THE FACILITIES ARE THERE FOR YOUR BENEFIT — IT'S UP TO YOU TO MAKE USE OF THEM . .

Plate 1 (cont.)   Breast self-examination

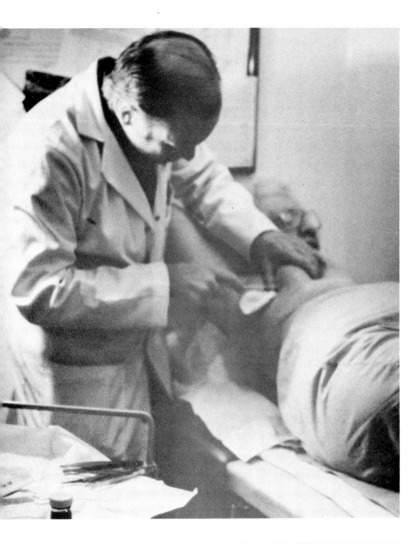

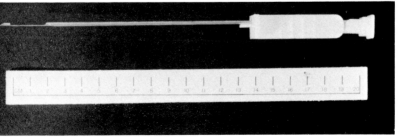

Plate 2   Needle biopsy

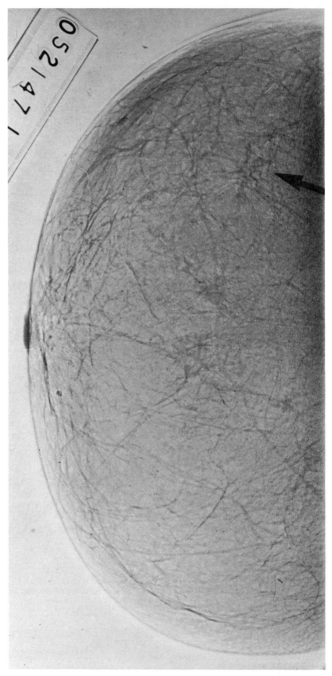

Plate 3 Mammogram of the breast of a woman with widespread breast can
producing anaemia as a result of infiltration of bone marrow. The arrow points
a very small primary cancer which was not detectable by palpation

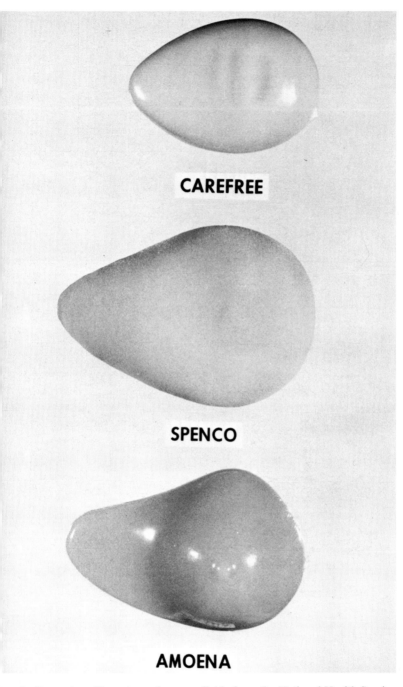

CAREFREE

SPENCO

AMOENA

ate 4   Examples of breast prostheses available from the National Health Service
in the United Kingdom

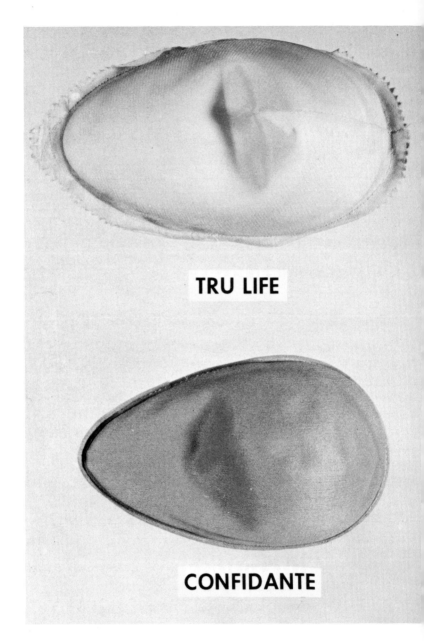

TRU LIFE

CONFIDANTE

Plate 4 (cont.)   Examples of breast prostheses

The course of breast cancer

carcinoma of the breast may disseminate to the vital organs at any point from when it is too small to be detected clinically until the tumour is many centimetres in diameter. Much current research work is involved in attempts to predict accurately the biological behaviour of individual cancers and to try and refine the information that may be achieved from 'grading' the tumour according to the degree of histological differentiation.

Staging of breast cancer

Before proceeding to surgery when cancer is suspected it is essential to define as accurately as possible the clinical stage of the disease. The staging system recommended by the International Union Against Cancer (UICC) is illustrated in Table 4 and a comparison with the Manchester classification is shown in Table 5. In the simplest terms, Stage I disease is confined to the breast, whereas in Stage II disease the regional lymph nodes are thought to be involved by cancer. Only these two stages are considered 'curable' (operable). Stage III or locally advanced disease is usually treated by radiotherapy and Stage IV disease, with obvious distant dissemination, is treated with some form of sytemic therapy as described in Chapter 9. As an aid to staging of the disease a chest X-ray should be carried out to look for lung metastases or involvement of the membranes around the lungs. Skeletal radiology or scintigraphy should be carried out to search for bone metastases and, although rarely helpful, some form of biochemical and haematological screen should be performed to detect evidence of liver or bone marrow involvement.

Table 4. *Clinical staging of breast cancer (UICC)*

Tumour status

T_0	No palpable tumour.
T_1	Tumour 2 cm or less with no fixation.
T_2	Tumour more than 2 cm but less than 5 cm with no fixation.
T_3	Tumour more than 5 cm maximum diameter. (For T_{1-3} suffix A implies no attachment to underlying muscles. B implies such attachment).
T_4	Tumour of any size with either fixation to chest wall or ulceration of skin.

Status of lymph nodes

N_0	No palpable axillary nodes.
N_{1A}	Palpable axillary nodes not considered to contain tumour.
N_{1B}	Palpable nodes thought to contain tumour.
N_2	Nodes greater than 2 cm or fixed to one another and deep structures.
N_3	Supraclavicular or infraclavicular nodes.

Distant metastases

M_0	No clinically apparent distant metastases.
M_1	Distant metastases obvious.

Table 5. *Comparison between the 'Manchester' and UICC classification*

Stage I	T_{1A}	N_0	M_0
	T_{2A}	N_0	
Stage II	T_0	N_1	
	T_{1A}	N_1	M_0
	T_{2A}	N_1	
Stage III	T_3	$N_{0,1,2}$	
	$T_{0,1,2}$	N_2	M_0
	T_{1B}, T_{2B}	$N_{0,1,2}$	
	T_4	$N_{0,1,2}$	
Stage IV	Any T	N_3 or	M_1

8

Surgery

A change in emphasis

Until about 20 years ago the objectives of surgery for primary breast cancer were easy to define, to wit, the clearance of every last cancer cell from the breast and the regional lymph nodes. Similarly, the choice of surgery was simple and non-controversial, as the classical radical mastectomy was thought to achieve these objectives and the mutilation and morbidity that followed this procedure was considered an acceptable price to pay for the life of the woman. These days it is no longer that simple, either to define the objectives of surgery or to select the most appropriate procedure.

As described in Chapter 1, any improvement in survival statistics achieved by the radical mastectomy between the 1930s and the 1950s could be ascribed to better methods of selection by excluding those cases from surgery who were doomed to rapid local recurrence and death. Over the last 20 years the survival statistics following radical local treatment have remained stubbornly constant, approximately 50 per cent at ten years.

In recent years new evidence has accumulated suggesting that breast cancer cells gain direct access to the bloodstream and then to the vital organs early in the course of tumour development. Furthermore, tumour cells that reach the lymph nodes are not necessarily trapped there but can either traverse the lymph nodes intact or bypass the lymph nodes via lympho-venous communications. In addition, the lymph nodes themselves may be regarded as actively hostile to the proliferation of tumour cells, owing to the inherent antitumour activity of the lymphocytes and histiocytes that are present in large numbers. With the assimilation of these findings from basic cancer research, a new understanding concerning the biological nature of breast cancer has evolved. It is suggested that if the lymph nodes draining a breast cancer are uninvolved, this may represent a favourable tumour–host balance with the patient's natural resistance to the spread of the cancer remaining intact, and it was even considered until quite recently that the removal or irradiation of these uninvolved lymph nodes might be potentially harmful to the patient. On the other hand, if the lymph nodes are involved with tumour, this probably indicates that the disease is widely disseminated owing to the exhaustion of the natural resistance to the cancer. Treatment of the axillary (underarm) nodes in these instances might be important for symptomatic relief but would be unlikely to increase the cure rate.

Over the last 10–20 years several clinical trials have compared various radical forms of treatment with various more conservative approaches. In general no one form of treatment has been demonstrated to be superior to any other as far as survival is concerned, but all trials have consistently demonstrated the very poor outlook connected with involvement of the axillary nodes. To summarize the currently held view, therefore, it is believed that except in rare instances the involved axillary node is not a nidus for tertiary spread of the disease but merely symptomatic that the disease is already systemic. Secondly, the outcome of treatment is not determined by the extent of the original operation but by the extent of undetectable metastases in vital organs present at the time of diagnosis.

Surgery in the 1980s

What then are the objectives of surgery for primary breast cancer in the 1980s?

1 In selected cases, where the disease is confined to the breast (see Chapter 3) surgery alone, either by simple

mastectomy or wide local excision of the local tumour, might be sufficient to achieve cure.

2 In all other cases surgery has an important role in achieving local control of the disease so that even if the woman subsequently dies of metastatic breast cancer at least she is not distressed by a painful, infected, and ulcerated chest wall.

3 Determining the pathological stage of the involvement of the axilla and perhaps the internal mammary lymph nodes is now considered an essential role of the first surgical approach to the disease, in order to determine accurately the outlook for the woman. The importance of this becomes obvious when considering adjuvant systemic therapy, as described in the next chapter.

4 It is likely to become increasingly important to have as large a sample of tumour as possible for further histological and biological assessments. It has already been described in Chapter 3 how the histological differentiation of the primary tumour can be a guide to outlook, but more important than that are recent developments in the assessment of the biological properties of the primary cancer. For example, measurement of the oestradiol receptor (see page 22) within the tumour will help clinicians select appropriate therapy should the disease relapse, or perhaps guide the clinician in his choice of adjuvant systemic therapy following mastectomy.

1 Surgery for cure†

The classical Halsted *radical mastectomy* involved removing the whole breast, the underlying pectoral muscles in continuity with the axillary contents up to the so-called apex of the axilla, where the axillary artery and vein pass over the first rib (see Figure 2, page 18). A more radical extension of this procedure involved lifting a flap of the chest wall overlying

† See also Chapter 3, section 'Structures removed at surgery'.

the internal mammary lymph nodes, which were then removed as a separate procedure (the so-called super-radical
mastectomy). Even assuming that some cancers are confined
to the breast and regional lymph nodes alone, then the same
objectives may be achieved with much less surgical damage
by leaving the pectoralis major muscle intact and clearing
the axilla in continuity with the breast, facilitated by removing the pectoralis minor alone. This so-called modified (Patey)
mastectomy is increasing in popularity throughout the world
and allows women to wear swimming costumes and low neck-
lines in the confidence that their deformity can easily be dis-
guised by an external prosthesis.

However, if it is assumed that where the lymph nodes are
involved the patient has a high statistical probability of having
widely disseminated disease at diagnosis, then radical clearance of the regional lymph nodes with the objective of cure
is analogous to 'shutting the stable door after the horse has
bolted'. With this idea in mind there has been something of
a reaction against radical surgery over the last ten years, with
many clinicians arguing that, in those cases that are truly
curable, cure could equally well be achieved by *simple mastectomy* alone, leaving the axilla untouched, or wide local
excision of the primary tumour, perhaps supplemented by
postoperative radiotherapy. There is certainly a worldwide
momentum developing towards breast conservation which
will be discussed later in this chapter.

2 *Surgery for local control of breast cancer*

Assuming that only about 30 per cent of the most favourable
cases selected for mastectomy will be cured, then perhaps
the most pragmatic approach for the surgeon to adopt is to
aim at local control of the disease. Unfortunately, whatever
form of local therapy is used, there seems to be a hard core
of cases, ranging from 5 to 10 per cent, in which local recurrence eventually catches up with the patient. From a variety

of prospective clinical trials the following conclusions can be reached concerning the incidence of local recurrence.

1 Radical mastectomy followed by radiotherapy is equivalent to simple mastectomy followed by radiotherapy.
2 Radical mastectomy alone has a higher incidence of local recurrence than radical mastectomy followed by radiotherapy.
3 Simple mastectomy alone has a higher incidence of local recurrence than simple mastectomy followed by immediate radiotherapy.
4 Delayed radiotherapy following either simple or radical mastectomy is likely to produce adequate control in the majority of cases when recurrence occurs.
5 The more extensive the primary surgery, the more difficult is the rehabilitation of the woman; in particular the incidence of severe lymphoedema (swelling caused by excess fluid) of the arm is highest after radical surgery combined with postoperative radiotherapy and lowest after conservative surgery alone.

On the basis of these observations, the surgeon today is faced with a considerable dilemma. Should he be more concerned about avoiding the extreme anxiety experienced by a woman who observes that her primary treatment has failed, or should he consider the other side of the coin and look at the benefits of the more conservative approach which speed up the rehabilitation of the patient and reduce the incidence of lymphoedema of the arm to a minimum? At present I personally favour a simple mastectomy with dissection of the lower part of the axilla (see below) with postoperative radiotherapy if the axilla is pathologically involved, but I believe that no surgeon should have fixed ideas and should be prepared to modify his primary treatment strategy as the results of long-term clinical trials become available.

3 *Staging the disease*

As already described, the most important variable affecting outlook in a patient presenting with primary breast cancer is the pathological status of the regional lymph nodes. Furthermore, the degree of involvement of these lymph nodes allows us to define sub-groups according to outlook. At the worst end of the scale, generally speaking, if there is involvement above the level of the pectoralis minor, or alternatively if four or more of the nodes that are sampled contain tumour, then it can be judged that 80 per cent of these women will be dead within ten years of mastectomy. Since the development of effective cytotoxic chemotherapy regimens for the advanced disease (see next Chapter), a rational approach has been to introduce these agents following mastectomy in those patients identified as being at greatest risk as judged by involvement of the axillary nodes. For this reason it is vitally important to take a sample from the axilla, i.e. determine the stage of the disease, at the time of primary surgery. A complete clearance of the underarm contents would, of course, be guaranteed to produce the best evidence required and this remains a compelling argument in favour of a modified radical mastectomy. But, as already stated, this radical dissection adds to the risk to postoperative lymphoedema. A suitable compromise favoured by many in the United Kingdom is a dissection limited to the lower third of the axilla, say below the level of the pectoralis minor, at the time of total mastectomy, as knowledge of the pathological status of the axilla higher than this level does not significantly help the surgeon to estimate the prognosis. In addition, many surgeons feel it is important to know the pathological status of the internal mammary nodes at the time of mastectomy, and complete their operation by dissecting out one or two nodes from the spaces between the first and second ribs.

4 *Sampling of the tumour*

In our momentum towards conservation of the breast, I think it would be a pity if opportunities were lost for taking a sample of the primary cancer for a fully scientific evaluation of its biological properties. Ideally about one gram of tumour should be available for assessment of the oestradiol receptor content of the tumour as a way of predicting its endocrine responsiveness (see Chapters 7 and 9). Apart from this important biological variable, there are many new laboratory techniques being developed which will eventually help us to type the cancer accurately and to be able to predict with greater precision its likelihood of dissemination and the sensitivity of the cancer cells to either endocrine or chemical treatment.

Breast conservation

Another issue, which is perhaps of more interest to the average woman than whether or not the mastectomy operation should be extended to her axilla, is the place of breast conservation following treatment for primary carcinoma. Contrary to the stereotype image, today's breed of surgeon is well aware of the psychological insult that may follow a mastectomy (see Chapter 10). Apart from the compassionate motive for preserving the breast, there is the widely held view that should the public be aware that a lump in the breast need not necessarily imply a mastectomy, women would present themselves earlier in the development of the disease.

There are a number of approaches which effectively conserve the breast or at least preserve the appearance of a relatively normal-looking appendage on the chest wall. The surgeon may remove all the breast tissue from under the skin, preserving the nipple and filling the cavity with a silicone implant, the so-called subcutaneous mastectomy. Alternatively, following a local excision of the tumour, the residual breast and lymphatic fields can be treated by radical radiotherapy. Even more conservatively, the surrounding breast tissue and regional nodes can be treated by radical radiotherapy alone, following diagnosis via needle biopsy or aspiration cytology of the tumour. Treatment of the tumour alone is considered inadequate because, although the disease may appear to be affecting one site within the breast, in 40 per cent or more of cases it is known to represent a multifocal change within the whole breast tissue, with other areas of premalignant or frankly malignant change.

There are many encouraging reports from uncontrolled studies, conducted in Paris and Boston, Mass., which suggest that these conservative measures are entirely adequate and equivalent to treatment that involves mastectomy. In spite of this, extreme caution is urged in the interpretation of these data because inevitably in uncontrolled studies there will have been an element of selection, with perhaps only the most favourable cases being entered into the series. Nonetheless, there is a sufficient body of evidence to suggest that this approach is worth serious consideration and a number of prospective clinical trials are now in progress in the United States of America, Italy, and the United Kingdom to judge whether breast conservation is entirely safe. The one controlled study with adequate follow-up that has so far been reported was conducted by the Guy's Hospital Breast Unit. The authors of this study again urge caution, as those patients with Stage II disease treated conservatively demonstrated a higher incidence of local recurrence and an accelerated death rate than those treated conventionally. Some additional useful information came from the Guy's Breast Clinic Study in that it drew attention to the fact that only a small proportion of women with carcinoma of the breast are suitable for local excision and even in this group the cosmetic results left a lot to be desired.

It would, therefore, be quite wrong at the present time to publicize widely to the general public that breast conservation is feasible as it would inevitably lead to a bitter disappointment for the majority of women with the disease. At the present state in the evolution of treatment for carcinoma of the breast surgeons and patients alike would probably agree that cure is more important than contour, but at the same time surgeons should be encouraged to enter patients into prospective studies to evaluate breast conservation scientifically.

Conclusion

Twenty or thirty years ago my surgical colleagues had a very simple task when faced with a woman with early breast cancer. With no argument, radical mastectomy was the treatment of choice. From the preceding discussion, the reader might be excused if he or she was more confused than before. In fact the surgeon himself has an extremely difficult task in choosing the appropriate procedure for each case, and I believe that a number of the strategies available can achieve the same objectives. Perhaps for this reason women should start becoming more involved in the decision-making process. Therefore, provided the initial therapeutic approach achieves local control of the disease, adequate sampling of the tumour and of the axilla, and allows rapid rehabilitation of the patient, the precise details are not all that important. What *is* important though is that all clinicians should continue to keep an open mind, enter patients into clinical trials, and be prepared to change their policies as the results of these studies become available over the next ten years or so. Rigid adherence to inherited dogma will do nothing to advance the cause of science or the care of the patient.

9

Complementary therapy for primary breast cancer

Until relatively recently the responsibility for the management of early breast cancer rested entirely in the hands of the surgeon. Recognition that surgery alone does not have the entire answer for carcinoma of the breast has initiated a laudable progression towards a multidisciplinary approach in the management of the disease. As a result many surgeons these days set aside a short period each week for combined clinics with their radiotherapy/oncology colleagues, where they can discuss the management of breast cancer patients. Although this team approach is to be commended, treatment by committee has its disadvantages, and I personally believe that the surgeon should still remain the specialist of primary referral for patients with breast lumps, and should still retain the responsibility for continuity of care.

Treatment that is complementary to primary surgery can be considered under two broad headings; first, postoperative radiotherapy with the objective of improving local control of the disease, and secondly, adjuvant systemic therapy, the object of which is to destroy hidden foci of the cancer already established within the vital organs.

Postoperative radiotherapy

It is beyond dispute that whatever the extent of the original surgery for primary breast cancer, the addition of radiotherapy to the chest wall and the regional lymph node fields improves the degree of local control of the disease. Nevertheless, there is still some argument as to whether this additional treatment should be delivered as a preventive measure for the sake of the 20–30 per cent of women who will ultimately develop local or regional recurrence following surgery alone, or whether treatment should be delayed and be given therapeutically only when recurrence has been confirmed. Probably the correct answer to this dilemma is to be increasingly selective in judging which patients should be referred for postoperative radiotherapy, i.e. choose those who have the greatest risk of local recurrence following surgery alone. A reasonable policy to adopt would be to choose those patients with large primary tumours, particularly if they demonstrated a highly undifferentiated pattern on histological examination. In addition, those patients having less than a full surgical clearance of the underarm region, and who demonstrate pathological involvement of the lymph node sample, would probably benefit from postoperative radiotherapy to prevent uncontrollable axillary recurrence, even though such treatment would be unlikely to influence long-term survival. When patients have been referred for treatment, it is conventional for the radiotherapist to irradiate the chest wall and regional lymph nodes in the internal mammary chain, the depressions under and over the collar-bone, and the axilla.

The side-effects of radiotherapy have been grossly exaggerated in the past. Many old wives' tales have been passed on, for example as a result of the experience of someone's grandmother treated by radium needles in the years between the world wars. There is absolutely no truth in the beliefs that radiotherapy to the chest wall causes the hair to fall out, or that it makes the patient radioactive and therefore a danger to her immediate family! It is true that some degree of malaise and nausea may be experienced, but it is difficult to separate out the psychosomatic from the organic explanation for the symptoms. Fair-skinned, red-haired women are more likely to get severe skin reactions, but these are becoming less and less common with modern techniques.

Perhaps the main problem with radiotherapy is the inconvenience to the patient, particularly if elderly, of paying three visits a week to the hospital for up to six weeks. Very rarely excessive fibrous tissue, radiation fibrosis, of the apex of the lung may develop, producing a dry cough or shortness of breath, as a late sequel of the treatment, but again with glancing fields and supervoltage techniques, this can be easily avoided. Radiotherapy to the axilla following a radical dissection is not prescribed because of the severe lympho-edema of the arm that can result from this combined approach. There seems little doubt that regional radiotherapy can produce long-term effects on the cellular mechanism of immunity as judged by depression of the lymphocyte count, as well as interference with other somewhat esoteric mechanisms of immunity. In the recent past this was thought to be a serious contraindication to radiotherapy, as immunity was thought to have an important role to play in the control of micro-metastases. Although these mechanisms have an undoubted role in the resistance to the development and spread of experimental cancers in rats and mice, there is very little evidence from human studies that the depression of the lymphocyte count induced by ionizing radiation is of clinical relevance.

With prospects of breast conservation being seriously considered, new radiotherapy techniques are being evolved. It is interesting to remember that Sir Geoffrey Keynes from St. Bartholomew's Hospital was treating breast cancer by the insertion of radium needles in the 1930s; there has been a renewed interest in so-called interstitial radiation with the use of radioactive irridium wire threaded through the tumour. Using these techniques radiotherapists in Paris and Boston are now producing excellent cosmetic results in spite of extremely high doses of radiotherapy localized to the tumour site.

Adjuvant systemic therapy

As discussed in previous chapters, it is likely that in about 70 per cent of women subjected to mastectomy for apparently localized carcinoma of the breast, blood-borne dissemination of cancer cells, capable of multiplying to form a secondary growth elsewhere, has already occurred. Untreated, these progress to contribute to the death of the patient up to 20 years after surgery. It would seem reasonable, therefore, to hope that some form of treatment to other systems of the body ('systemic' treatment), directed at the elimination of these micro-metastases would lead to the improvement in survival figures following local treatment for 'early' carcinoma of the breast. The types of systemic treatment that are used are endocrine and cytotoxic therapy.

Because all such treatments have unwanted side-effects, with perhaps one or two exceptions (see below), it is generally accepted that some form of selection is necessary to predict that group of women most likely to develop distant metastases. In the last ten years or so there has been an enormous flurry of activity to try and improve on the accuracy of foretelling outlook achieved by simple clinical and pathological staging of the primary tumour (see page 53). Isotope scintigraphy of the skeleton and liver may occasionally pick up unsuspected metastases, and biochemical indices of invasion of the liver and bones may sometimes prove helpful. Nevertheless, the most efficient and reliable indicator of the presence of micro-metastases at the time of diagnosis is a careful pathological assessment of the contents of the axilla removed at the time of mastectomy. Most clinicians would now agree that trials of *toxic* systemic therapy should concentrate on the 'node-positive' group of patients following mastectomy, but where the systemic therapy is free of short-term or long-term side-effects, then perhaps all women with operable breast cancer might be considered for such complementary therapy.

Adjuvant endocrine therapy

The types of adjuvant endocrine therapy that have been evaluated in the past or are in the process of current evaluation are oophorectomy (removal of ovaries), irradiation of the ovaries, 'chemical adrenalectomy' (inhibition of the adrenal glands using corticosteroids), and anti-oestrogen therapy. A number of trials reported over the last 20 years have demonstrated that oophorectomy performed as a preventive measure, or ovarian ablation by radiotherapy for premenopausal women, induce a delay in the appearance of distant metastases for a number of years after mastectomy, but little or no long-term benefit as far as survival is concerned. This has led most specialists to withhold preventive removal of the ovaries because of the often distressing menopausal symptoms and the psychological insult that it inflicts. Nonetheless, a recent study from Toronto has suggested that removal of the ovaries combined with long-term treatment with corticosteroids may indeed produce significant improvements in survival as well as delay in the appearance of distant metastases.

Much current interest has been generated by the new group of drugs referred to as the anti-oestrogens, of which tamoxifen (Nolvadex) is perhaps the most effective and least toxic. This drug works by competing for the binding site on the oestradiol receptor (see Chapters 2 and 11). Two major trials are now underway in the United Kingdom to evaluate the 'gentle' drug as adjuvant systemic therapy for both node-positive and node-negative women.

Adjuvant chemotherapy

Chemotherapy for malignant disease would ideally exploit some property of malignant cells not shared with ordinary cells. As no such property is yet known, chemotherapy involves the use of agents known as cytotoxic drugs that damage all growing cells. The early trials of systemic chemotherapy following mastectomy used short courses of ankylating agents (drugs related to mustard gas) within the peri-operative and immediately postoperative period, with the expressed objective of destroying any cancer cells that were shed at the time of manipulation of the tumour during surgery. Although this mode of dissemination is now considered relatively unimportant, recent-results from a major Scandinavian trial have in fact demonstrated a 10 per cent improvement in survival at ten years post-mastectomy. Because of the relatively low toxicity of this approach such an apparently modest benefit is still worth the expense.

The majority of current trials of systemic chemotherapy are using combinations of cytotoxic drugs given in cycles at approximately monthly intervals for up to two years after mastectomy. This approach is based on the kinetic studies of cancer growth and aimed at destroying established metastases rather than circulating cancer cells. The pioneering experiences reported by the National Surgical Adjuvant Breast Project in the United States of America and the Tumour Institute in Milan show quite encouraging early results which in particular seem to benefit the premenopausal group of women. In spite of this, most specialists in this country would be hesitant to recommend the wholesale adoption of this approach until longer-term results are available. There are a number of cogent reasons for this apparent conservatism.

First of all the treatments are extremely toxic, leading to alopecia (loss of hair), nausea, and vomiting, as well as suppression of bone marrow function (production of blood cells and platelets) in a high proportion of cases. The treatment needs to be delivered by specialists who are not always available in busy surgical clinics. So far postmenopausal women have failed to respond and the question still remains open as to whether chemotherapy delayed until the appearance of distant metastases will acheive the same long-term result as immediate preventive chemotherapy following mastectomy. There is also a small nagging worry that the prolonged use of alkylating agents, which are themselves carcinogenic, in women who may yet live 10–20 years, may induce second cancers. Notwithstanding these reservations, the early results of the programmes of complementary systemic therapy are perhaps the single main cause for optimism in the whole subject of early carcinoma of the breast.

10

Psychosocial aspects of breast cancer and rehabilitation

Introduction

The breast should not be considered as a mere appendage of lactation, of no further use once the phase of childbearing is complete. The breast also has a role in sexual attraction, the maintenance of self-esteem, and body image, all of which may vary in importance with marital status, age, and current fashions in dress. Even a matronly, middle-aged woman values her breasts as reminders of her feminine role; and more than one obese, elderly mastectomy patient has mourned her loss when wishing to hug and comfort a weeping grandchild. Thus, a woman faced with the threat of mastectomy has to face the fear of mutilation with its psychological and social consequences, as well as the fear of cancer.

It is conventional to consider the psychological aspects of breast cancer as they affect the nine phases of progression of the disease from pre-detection until the terminal stage. These may be listed as follows:

1 Pre-detection
2 Post-detection/pre-diagnosis
3 The diagnostic and evaluation phase
4 Preoperative phase
5 Immediate post-mastectomy phase
6 Rehabilitation and psychological adjustment to mastectomy
7 The follow-up
8 The recurrent disease
9 The terminal phase

Pre-detection

Previously in this book I have argued the case for limited screening for high-risk populations and also for public health education to persuade women to carry out routine self-examination and to see their doctor as soon as possible after detection of the lump. Yet, in spite of this, and even if a screening clinic exists, reports have demonstrated that anything between 20 and 60 per cent of women invited to attend for pre-symptomatic diagnosis refuse the invitation, and similarly a number of surveys investigating the extent of the practice of routine self-examination have shown that it is only a very small minority of women who carry out this very simple and potentially life-saving manoeuvre.

An extremely simplistic explanation for these associated findings would be to ascribe them to ignorance on the part of the women due to inadequate public health education. To an extent this might be true as far as the quality rather than the quantity of public health education available is concerned. This is illustrated by the common sight at a specialist breast clinic of a large number of terrified young women complaining of pain in the breast who think they have cancer, yet, because of their age and symptomatology, almost certainly do not. At the other extreme, many older women will attend with a history of a lump in the breast, present for many months, who did not think it was anything to worry about because it *was not* painful. At this level it should be relatively easy to get through to young women at an impressionable age (perhaps as part of their school curriculum) that it is common to experience some discomfort and even pain in the breast before periods in the early years after the menarche, and at the same time to explain that all lumps detected in the breast should be reported immediately to the doctor. The advantages of prompt self-referral are easy to explain: three out of four lumps will be entirely innocent and rapid attention to these can do away with weeks of sleepless nights, whereas on the other hand for the women in the cancer age group prompt detection and treatment of a small breast cancer might increase the chances of cure.

Be that as it may, there is an enormous psychological barrier amongst women who are perfectly well educated about self-examination, screening, and the significance of breast lumps, and they may behave in what might be considered as an irrational manner. There is no denying the fact, therefore, that many women will not examine their own breasts *in case* they should find something, and similarly many women refuse the invitation to attend a screening clinic *in case* the doctors find something. Before remedial public health education can come to terms with this problem, more basic research on the psychodynamics of self-help is required.

Post-detection

Once a woman detects a lump in her breast there are, in broad general terms, two patterns of behaviour. The first may be described as impetuous, where without further thought, spurred on by fear, the woman seeks medical attention, and may be at the practitioner's surgery the morning after discovering the lump. At the other extreme there is the pattern of denial, in which the woman, having detected the lump, may defer reporting the symptoms to the doctor for intervals varying between a month to several years. Intuition might tell us that the first type of reaction is the more rational and relates to a higher intelligence as judged by educational attainment, yet this does not seem to be the case, according to a number of attitude surveys that have been published to date. When questioning the women whose behaviour pattern has been that of denial and delay, ignorance as to the significance of breast lumps hardly features as an explanation. In the majority of cases it is fear of confirmation that they have breast cancer that leads to procrastination. The fear not only relates to the life threat but to the disruption of their life pattern. It is not surprising, therefore, that a disproportionate number of these women have an obsessional or organized behaviour trait. Surprisingly enough, fear of mastectomy itself seldom features as an explanation for the delay and there is very little evidence to justify the commonly held belief that public knowledge of the possibility of breast conservation therapy for cancer would result in earlier presentation of the disease.

The diagnostic and evaluation phase

Once a woman with breast symptoms has been referred to the surgeon, it is a reasonable assumption that she believes that she has breast cancer until reassured otherwise. It is not surprising, therefore, that by all measurable criteria women attending breast clinics and awaiting the results of diagnostic procedures are suffering from very intense anxiety. Apart from the formal psychological tests for anxiety, a few questions to the woman about disturbance of sleep, appetite, and mood will reveal the torment that she is suffering. It is very important, therefore, that the surgeon should recognize this problem and adopt an open approach with the patient and discuss the likelihood of the symptoms being related to cancer and arrive at a definitive diagnosis as quickly as possible. For this reason aspiration of cysts and outpatient diagnosis of solid lumps by cytology or needle biopsy, as described in Chapter 6, are not only efficient from the management point of view, but humane in removing the doubt and uncertainty in the woman's mind as quickly as possible.

The preoperative phase

Once a diagnosis of cancer has been firmly established and the patient's admission arranged for mastectomy, the anxiety of uncertainty has been removed, but the woman now has to face the fear of what to many is still a life-threatening operation and the disruption of her life resulting from a week or two in hospital. This problem is acutely severe amongst women with young children, and may necessitate the husband taking time off work, and in single-parent families, who may require help from the social work department. Reassurance from the surgeon that the operation these days is relatively minor may help with some of the patient's fears, but probably the kindest approach is to arrange the admission and operation as quickly as possible, not because the management of breast cancer is an emergency, but to shorten as much as possible this episode of threat and crisis.

The immediate post-mastectomy phase

It is a curious phenomenon for those not experienced in the management of the mastectomy patient to witness the period of relative euphoria in the first few days after the mastectomy. This probably relates to the fact that all uncertainty and ambiguity has been removed, and that they have come through an operation which, as explained before, is still considered a major life-threat to the majority of the lay public. Many women will also be pleasantly surprised by the rapidity with which they regain their arm movement, and some may even be surprised that the extent of mutilation, particularly following simple or modified radical procedures, is less than they anticipated. They also eagerly anticipate the return to their family and have not yet begun to reconsider the life-threat of the cancer itself. It is essential to exploit this short period to hasten physical rehabilitation by encouraging active arm movements and by the earliest possible prescription of a temporary prosthesis. Whilst the sutures are still in or the wound is not fully healed, most women cannot tolerate the heavy, permanent external prosthesis, but can rapidly regain their confidence and make themselves attractive in their nighties by wearing a soft, lightweight prosthesis under their bra.

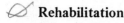

Rehabilitation

Rehabilitation following discharge from hospital after a mastectomy can be sub-divided under two headings – physical and psychological. The first is relatively simple; the second is complex to say the least.

Physical rehabilitation

As the use of the classical radical mastectomy declines in popularity in the United Kingdom the problem of the stiff shoulder following mastectomy has almost disappeared. Provided that women are reassured very early on that they are not going to damage the wound or disrupt the sutures, they are usually willing to tolerate the modest amount of discomfort that goes along with encouraging them to use their shoulder to the maximum. Physiotherapists, nurses, and surgeons should encourage active rather than passive exercises, so that by the time the woman has left the hospital she should be able to brush the back of her hair and do up zips at the back of her dress. Full movement of the shoulders can be encouraged by the simple exercise of 'walking up the wall' with the hands so that eventually both arms are stretched right above the head with the palms symmetrically placed against the wall. The use of such exercises will probably also reduce the incidence of lymphoedema that may follow a full surgical removal of the underarm contents, but in addition a woman may occasionally need elastic bandaging or elevation of the arm whilst she sleeps.

A much greater problem connected with physical rehabilitation, which also has profound influence on the psychological rehabilitation, is the prescription of an adequate external prosthesis. Most surgeons, nurses, and for that matter appliance officers are woefully ignorant about the types and variety of external prostheses that are available. It must be categorically stated that any surgeon can prescribe *any* prosthesis, which may be replaced at *any* interval irrespective of cost, if in the surgeon's opinion the prescription is justified. Plate 4 illustrates some of the wide variety of appliances that are available. According to their weight, shape, and quality of adherence to the chest wall different types may suit different women at different times. Yet the conventional practice is for the surgeon to countersign a form that merely states: 'mastectomy/prosthesis', and leave the rest to the appliance officer in the hospital.

Psychological rehabilitation

The period of postoperative euphoria rapidly dissipates and women become psychologically most vulnerable at about two to three months after mastectomy. Thereafter there appears to be a period of shock and denial. Then, when denial is no longer possible to sustain, a period of anxiety supervenes, which, again, may be recognized by insomnia, anorexia, and mood changes. Anxiety is usually replaced by a period of anger or guilt and this may be transferred to the husband or surgeon. Then, a period of depression may follow, particularly if the mastectomy has proved a threat to valued activities, which, of course, includes sexual relationships with their partner. Even when this is not a problem interference with activities such as swimming or the wearing of fashionable clothes may be reason enough to prolong the depressive phase. Finally, after a variable length of time a coping style is arrived at in the majority of cases. This coping style may be of stoic acceptance or frank denial, but it must be emphasized that 70–80 per cent of women have sufficient resilience on their own to arrive at a solution that best fits them for continuing to live their life as they choose. Nonetheless, a number of studies in this country have demonstrated that between one to two years after a mastectomy about 20–30 per cent of women have residual psychological and sexual problems. However, to keep this in perspective, it must be remembered that women in the breast cancer age group may also be exposed to other stressful life events, such as bereavement, problems with teenage children, and problems with unemployment of the breadwinner within the family. In fact, controlled studies have demonstrated that about 10 per cent of age-matched women over a period of one to two years will also develop serious psychological and sexual problems. This still leaves an excess of 15–20 per cent of mastectomy patients who probably need some form of additional help above that which they can provide themselves.

It is at this point that the husband's positive role must be emphasized. I strongly believe that the husband should be involved in all stages right through from the diagnosis to the post-mastectomy phase. The husband often feels guilt himself, but he needs to be reassured on this score and urged to demonstrate his affection and to seek intimacy with his wife. Often the woman feels that she will cease to be sexually attractive to her partner, and because of this fear of rejection or revulsion, she may refuse to undress and avoid sexual encounters and thus institute a self-fulfilling prophecy. Yet in the majority of cases with adequate reassurance it is found that the stress of mastectomy may establish additional bonds of affection and mutual support that will further cement a marriage. Without a husband or significant partner, the mastectomy patient is particularly vulnerable and these women, together with those who have pre-existing psychological problems, need to be carefully watched for the detection of serious psychological morbidity that needs professional intervention.

The follow-up phase

Once the woman has learnt to cope with the mastectomy and the threat of cancer, each follow-up visit to the surgeon re-awakens dormant fears. 'What will they find this time?' may be the predictable reaction prior to each visit. Furthermore, each new ache and pain, as with the super-imposition of osteoarthritis as the woman ages, may be interpreted as a symptom of recurrent disease. Adjuvant systemic therapy will be a constant reminder that the woman is 'not well', and if this additional therapy carries with it toxic side-effects, then these may contribute to or prolong the natural history of the emotional adjustment to the mastectomy.

Recognition of recurrence

Perhaps the most difficult phase for a woman to cope with is the recognition of treatment failure by the appearance of local or distant metastases. As these commonly appear many years after the mastectomy, it is a shattering experience once more to have to adjust to the threat of death and mutilation. If one then adds to the woman's psychological trauma treatment such as removal of the ovaries and cytotoxic chemotherapy, one might predict that the load would be too great and that the majority of women would 'crack up' completely. Very little valid work has been conducted in this phase of the natural history of breast cancer, but I have formed the strong clinical impression that powerful denial mechanisms are once more triggered off and the woman becomes curiously dispassionate as if observing her bodily processes, symptoms, and therapy from a detached viewpoint.

Coming to terms with death

There comes a time eventually when the clinician wishes to withhold further active therapy and recognizes that the expectation of life is now limited to months rather than years. Once again at this stage the husband or significant partner should be involved in the discussions, but the clinician has not discharged his responsibility merely by explaining to the next of kin that death is imminent.

Remedial activity

From the above it can be judged that there is a long and

painful catalogue of psychological morbidity associated with breast disease. It is one of the privileges of dealing with these patients to recognize the incredible natural resources for coping that exist amongst the majority of women. But that aside, at all phases, quality of care could be improved to reduce the stresses involved. The mere recognition of the psychological sequelae of mastectomy by husbands and by all professional groups caring for the women, and a sensitive handling of the patient at each stage can go a long way to alleviating some of the stress. Apart from good doctoring and good nursing, two alternative strategies can be considered.

First, there are the volunteer groups of women, many of whom have had mastectomy themselves, such as the Mastectomy Association in the United Kingdom and the The Reach to Recovery Program in the United States of America; secondly, specialist nurses are now being recruited into many of the breast clinics in this country, who are known as Mastectomy Counsellors. Whatever strategy is evolved, I think it should be scientifically evaluated as natural coping mechanisms do exist in the majority of women, and it is at least conceivable that outside interference by well-meaning lay and professional groups may disturb the natural cycle of adjustment.

11

The role of the nurse-counsellor

Sylvia Denton

Introduction

The many women who have to face the fact that they have breast cancer not only have to contend with the reality of a life-threatening disease, but also with treatment which presents a threat to their feminine identity and feeling of well-being both within their family and the society in which they move.

The first symptoms of the disease are frequently found whilst a woman is feeling quite well, adding to her sense of unreality. On more than one occasion patients under my care have said: 'I feel as if I am dreaming all that is happening'. Thus, fear of disease and fear of deformity have to be faced by the patient, and those helping with her care must recognize these facts and assist her to draw on her own emotional resources to establish a secure strategy for coping with these fears.

Studies demonstrate that breast cancer treated by mastectomy may cause between 20 and 40 per cent of women to suffer a depressive illness. This bare statistic over-simplifies what is the end-result of a complex series of reactions and adjustments. The nurse-counsellor helping to care for patients with breast cancer may observe a vast range of reactions to this disease, the woman's emotions often changing with the passage of time, commonly eventually resulting in the development of a way of coping that is 'comfortable' to her. This natural sequence may require outside help, but help which should ideally be adapted by the professionals within the service to the patient's needs as time passes. This latter point is of great importance: the patient should always feel she is in control of what is happening to her and thus 'pace' the service offered.

The nurse-counsellor should have knowledge of counselling skills: Gaynor Nurse states that 'counselling is seen by some nurses as an integral part of their ordinary work, a function which may even be written into their job description'.

As a nurse-counsellor helping to care for the patient with breast cancer, I see my objective as providing a service which may offer emotional and practical support, assisting the patient to achieve her optimum potential for physical and psychological rehabilitation. With sufficient tact and a modicum of skill a relationship may rapidly be established between the patient and her nurse, enabling her to express her doubts and fears and to explore possible solutions to her problems. Knowledge of current treatment for breast cancer, together with information regarding prostheses, clothing, and provision for care within other agencies, such as the social services, charities, and other medical disciplines, is essential before a nurse attempts counselling. This knowledge should extend to the services provided within the community, for it is only when the patient emerges from the hospital gates upon discharge that she faces the realities of life again with the 'cocoon' of the hospital and the supportive 'feminine' environment of the ward.

The nurse-counsellor should endeavour to understand and appreciate the roles of ward staff, clinic staff, community nursing and medical personnel, and constantly be aware how best she can assist within this established framework. It is necessary for the nurse-counsellor to be able to recognize when her role should terminate and another discipline take over, and when the patient requires more specialist treatment or help, an obvious example being that of referral for psychiatric advice.

It is also of prime importance that the nurse be able to recognize when to terminate regular contact with the patient when the patient's own strategies for coping have become sufficiently well developed. To perpetuate professional contact on a regular basis prevents the patient from feeling she is able to cope on her own, thus singling her out as 'unwell'. At the same time it is advisable to leave some line of contact intact, such as an invitation to telephone. It is assumed that prior to this break a good enough relationship would have been established between the patient and the nurse to enable the patient to feel at liberty to contact the nurse if necessary.

Patients often see the nursing and medical staff as concerned solely for their physical well-being and they may be very reluctant initially to talk of their emotional problems. Equally, nurses and doctors may be so ill-prepared or even unwilling to concern themselves with patients' emotional reactions and social problems associated with their disease, that either one or both inhibit the formation of lines of communication.

Education on the subject of cancer may also be seen as part of the nurse-counsellor's role, for ignorance helps to promote fear, which is often exaggerated by the media making the patient more aware of the problems and questions surrounding their disease, rather than providing any reassurance. The counsellor must keep herself aware of current popular journalism and keep an eye on the television schedules so as to anticipate the distress that may be created by an incomplete understanding of articles and programmes.

The pattern of counselling

It must be emphasized that at the present time there is no routine service available for counselling in the majority of hospitals. What I am about to describe is a service that has evolved in a pilot study conducted in the Department of Surgery at King's College Hospital Medical School, thanks to the generosity of the Cancer Research Campaign and Marks and Spencers Limited.

Breast cancer: the facts

The nurse-counsellor attends the outpatients clinic, where needle biopsy is performed under local anaesthetic for women presenting with suspicious breast lumps. She is also present when the patient is informed of the diagnosis. This understandably is a traumatic experience for the woman regardless of whether or not she expected a diagnosis of cancer, and often very little verbal exchange occurs between patient and nurse at this stage. Nonetheless, a relationship should start to build up and the patient can receive comfort from someone with whom she can talk, and upon whose shoulder she may cry. The nurse here can give comfort just by her presence and understanding silence, allowing the patient to set the pace for development of the liaison. Names and telephone numbers can be exchanged and arrangements made for admission to hospital and prior to this, if convenient for the patient and desired by her, a home visit arranged. It is on this home visit that much is achieved as the patient often has many questions to ask, feeling more at ease in her own home. Relatives and friends may be present and they are encouraged to partake in the interview, for this is a 'family disease', every member having to adapt to its impact on the woman, whether she is a grandmother, sister, wife, daughter, or good friend.

The patient is seen on admission to the ward before her operation. It is again important not to probe too deeply so that the patient can set the pace of the interview and indicate what is important to her and what she wants to discuss. The word 'cancer' is used: we feel that the true diagnosis should be given and discussed with tact and empathy, thus eliminating the need to use euphemisms and begin the game of pretence. Further explanations are sometimes needed about practical details such as the general routine for the operation and an explanation of the wound drainage equipment that will be *in situ* when the patient recovers from anaesthesia. Patients also often want to know about stitches and to be given information about their appearance after the operation. In times of stress these things are often explained but very soon forgotten, so the message needs to be reinforced at subsequent interviews.

After operation the patient is seen as soon as possible and this is the time when the nurse can begin to give practical as well as emotional support. The subject of breast prostheses is introduced to the patient during the postoperative period in hospital. Prostheses should be introduced with care as some patients experience shock or even revulsion on seeing for the first time the prosthesis that has to become part of her underwear. When selecting a permanent prosthesis, it is very important that this is the patient's personal choice from the range of prostheses available to her and that she should feel confident when wearing it. This confidence can only be gained if the prosthesis both feels and looks good to the woman herself.

Discussion with the patient in the ward may enable her to explore her feelings about self-image, and also whether she has been able to look at her scar. This is a very important first step, often causing profound dismay. If acceptable and desired by the patient, this step may be assisted by the nurse-counsellor being with the patient when she looks at the wound for the first time. A home visit is made with prior arrangement about two to three weeks after discharge from hospital. At this time the woman is usually beginning to settle back into her routine. Often her husband or a family member who may have stayed at home to be with her initially has returned to work and perhaps there are fewer neighbours and friends calling, thus this is the time for morbid thoughts and worries to emerge. At this stage the woman commonly welcomes the opportunity to talk and express these fears at a timely visit from a member of the health care team. Further visits are arranged according to the patient's needs and referrals to more specialist services or agencies as required. A link is always kept with the patient who is given the specialist-nurse's telephone number for use when a psychological or social crisis develops, or for the mundane prescription of a new prosthesis.

Breast cancer: the facts

Illustrative case histories

Reaction to the news that mastectomy is advised as treatment for breast cancer varies tremendously. Many women experience the fear of having cancer as their main worry; others experience the fear of losing their feminine identity. Others just feel that everything is going out of control. This latter group is illustrated by my first case history, an intelligent, well-educated woman of 53 years. She had just been told of the diagnosis of cancer in her breast and advised that mastectomy was indicated. In the midst of her shock and natural distress she firmly wagged her finger at the consultant and nurse saying: 'don't think mastectomy is a foregone conclusion for me' and got up to go. At a later date during an interview prior to mastectomy this reaction was discussed by her and the nurse. She had felt extreme shock, but beyond this she felt that she had lost control of what was happening to her. Taking her own decision was very much part of regaining apparent control over her life again. She was also experiencing other stresses – her marriage was unstable at that time. With time and discussion, she started to cope and decided to undergo mastectomy. Also, happily, her marital relationship became much better, her husband proving very supportive, and as time progressed adversity drew the couple closer together and, although still experiencing some difficulties, this patient feels her marriage is far happier. She returned to her work (a very responsible post), is coping well with life and enjoying amateur dramatics in her spare time. She has self-confidence and again feels in control of what is happening in her life.

Sometimes a woman finds the fact that she has cancer almost too much to bear and this may be seen to overtake other worries and problems such as feminine identity and the physical loss of the breast. One of my patients was a slight, very nervous woman of 58 years, widowed within the last year. She sought information and requested a truthful diagnosis, expressing no surprise when the diagnosis of cancer

86

was given. Her sister had also undergone mastectomy some ten years previously. When her fears were confirmed she became very distressed and expressed anxieties about cancer and its possible spread. Bone scans had revealed no obvious bone secondaries and the fact that postoperative radiotherapy might be required was explained. She had her mastectomy and because of pathological involvement of underarm lymph nodes it was necessary to give her radiotherapy. Throughout her stay in hospital and after discharge she often appeared to want to talk to the nurse-counsellor, and indeed, if feeling particularly low, would often telephone for a home visit. She was also referred to the psychiatrist for some help and she found this of great assistance. She explained that she felt dirty having cancer and withdrew into herself, not being able to go out and meet people. This withdrawal was gradually overcome, but it was six months before she felt able to return to her job as a domestic help. For a long time this woman was unable to look to any future for herself and became completely incapacitated by the idea of a further cancer, but with help and support, this is slowly being overcome and coped with and I anticipate this progress will continue.

Unhappily cancer sometimes enters the lives of young families. My third case history is about a woman 35 years old, with two young children of seven and five years. This patient discovered a lump in her breast and, as she explained later, with the encouragement of her husband, sought help immediately. Throughout these procedures and clinic visits, the husband was quietly present and plainly gave his wife much support. The couple appeared to draw together and, although obviously distressed, sought consolation by mutual support. The nurse-counsellor introduced herself to them, but, to begin with, it was obvious that to talk at length would have been an invasion of their privacy. Later, whilst on the ward, the wife welcomed the opportunity to talk and discuss her fears, as did her husband when they were visited at home by the nurse. This was obviously a very united family needing initially to draw into itself to be able to cope, and then later to look outwards and plan the future.

This latter case is probably illustrative of the majority of women, who either alone or with the support of a loving husband, have sufficient natural resources to come to terms with breast cancer. It is important that counselling should not officiously interfere with natural coping mechanisms.

12

The advanced disease: palliation and terminal care

It is important to emphasize what is meant by 'advanced' breast cancer. This term refers to the stages of the disease that we know from experience are incurable by conventional methods, and are most easily described by the Manchester Clinical Classification (see Table 5, page 54) as Stage III and Stage IV disease. Stage III represents locally advanced breast cancer unsuitable for mastectomy where although no obvious distant metastases may be detected on clinical examination, the outlook is so poor that it is a fair assumption that perhaps 95 per cent of these women are already suffering from established disseminated disease. Attempts at mastectomy are futile as far as saving life is concerned, and furthermore unwise from the point of view of palliation, as the disease will often rapidly recur within the scar, leaving a problem that is more difficult to control. These relatively rare cases are conventionally treated by radiotherapy and trials are underway to investigate the role of adjuvant systemic therapy as described in Chapter 9.

Stage IV breast cancer are those cases where the distant metastases are obvious, and where we know that the woman has a very limited expectation of life. It adds to the tragedy, therefore, if a hasty mastectomy is carried out on such a woman before an adequate assessment has been made to determine the exact extent of the disease.

Evaluation and staging

As in all branches of medicine a careful clinical history and examination are essential before considering therapy. The history from the patient may reveal breathlessness which might indicate leakage of fluid into the pleural cavity, or (lining around the lungs), the patient may complain of nausea, anorexia, and weight loss, which might imply metastases in the liver. Furthermore, weakness and lethargy, suggesting anaemia or hypercalcaemia (excess calcium in the blood, caused by secondaries in bone), may be present. The clinical examination is important for two reasons. The first, as already emphasized, is for accurate staging: the detection of lymph node enlargement or skin metastases beyond the region of the primary tumour and the axilla on the same side all indicate a poor outlook. The clinical detection of leakage of fluid into the pleural cavity or the palpation of an enlarged liver may be evidence of involvement of vital organs. It is equally important, however, in the advanced case to document carefully and measure all assessable symptoms so as to define the criteria of response that are to be used in judging whether or not the patient is responding to treatment. The importance of defining the criteria of response at the outset of therapy is expanded upon later in this chapter.

If the patient first comes to the specialist with advanced disease, histological confirmation is best achieved by needle biopsy of the primary growth. This is easily carried out in the outpatient clinic when the patient first attends, so that initial therapy can be conducted without an admission into hospital. If the recurrence of the disease is within the skeleton or the major organs in a patient who has previously had a mastectomy, then histological confirmation is probably not justified and an unequivocal chest X-ray or skeletal survey would be acceptable evidence on which to institute systemic therapy.

The diagnosis of metastases in the liver or cerebral hemispheres of the brain may occasionally be problematical. A clinically enlarged liver with abnormal findings on ultrasonography, or with deranged liver function tests, would probably be acceptable evidence of liver involvement. Evidence of raised pressure within the skull, localizing central nervous system signs, and focal abnormalities on computerized tomography scanning of the brain would suffice for the diagnosis of cerebral metastases. Whatever the extent of the disease judged by clinical examination, all patients should have a chest X-ray, skeletal scintigraphy, a full blood count, and a biochemical profile of the blood. In this way it is not uncommon to pick up 'silent' lung metastases, skeletal metastases, and evidence of bone marrow infiltration or hypercalcaemia.

Symptomatic palliation

When defining the objectives of treatment for advanced breast cancer, it should be remembered that all patients with Stage IV disease have a limited life expectancy irrespective of treatment. Therefore, of the two objectives – palliation of symptoms and prolongation of life – the main emphasis has to be given to improving the quality rather than the length of the patient's remaining life. Fortunately in most cases both objectives may be obtained from the same treatment strategy, but it should constantly be borne in mind that a point may be reached where aggressive active therapy diminishes the quality of life to a level where stubborn perseverance ceases to be humane. This consideration is part of the art rather than the science of medicine.

In many ways the treatment of a woman with advanced breast cancer can be very rewarding because most of the symptomatic problems are amenable to control, at least in the short term. Examples of problems and action required may be listed as follows.

Skeletal pain

If the pain is from a solitary bony metastasis, then complete relief of symptoms can be achieved in about 95 per cent of cases by a short course of localized radiotherapy. If the bone pain is more generalized, then it is essential that adequate analgesia is provided. It is conventional to start with simple drugs such as Distalgesic, or DF 118, and to progress through the more potent drugs, such as Diconal, until opiates are required. Heroin and morphine, combined with Largactil to prevent nausea, are conveniently prescribed as 'Brompton's mixture' and will provide complete analgesia in adequate dosage for intractable pain.

Breathlessness

Breathlessness (dyspnoea) is a common feature of advanced breast cancer as a result of malignant lung effusions. In almost all cases this problem is controllable by drainage of the fluid through a tube, followed by the introduction of cytotoxic drugs (usually alkalating agents) into the pleural cavity, which effectively destroy the malignant cells on the lung surface. Occasionally dyspnoea may result from a condition known as lymphangitis carcinomatosa, where the lymphatic channels within the lungs become widely infiltrated with cancer. This condition is much more difficult to treat, but some relief may be achieved by the use of corticosteroids.

Liver metastases

Liver metastases, if they are rapidly expanding, can produce severe pain, which may even mimic acute inflammation of the gall bladder. In addition, they often induce nausea, anorexia, and pruritis. Shrinkage of these secondaries can be achieved by giving high doses of corticosteroids or, alternatively, wide-field radiotherapy to the area of the liver.

Brain metastases

Cerebral metastases may produce severe headache and focal central nervous system signs that need urgent relief. Again, shrinkage of the secondaries can be achieved by dehydration therapy or by prescribing corticosteroids, in particular Dexamethazone. Radiotherapy to the brain may achieve significant palliation as well.

Anaemia from bone marrow infiltration

Two patterns of anaemia may result from the infiltration of the bone marrow by breast cancer: the 'aplastic' variety due to the massive replacement of the germinal cells responsible for the production of the red and white cells of the blood, or the 'leuco-erythroblastic' variety resulting from sensitivity of the stem cells, which differentiate to form blood cells, to products released from breast cancer cells within the marrow. Occasionally the anaemia is also associated with a life-threatening thrombocytopenia (reduction in the number of blood platelets). Blood transfusions and platelet transfusions may be required in the short term, but for longer-term control large doses of corticosteroids, androgen therapy, or chemotherapy using the vinca-alkaloids (which have a bone-marrow-sparing effect) may all be employed.

Hypercalcaemia

Hypercalcaemia, an excess of calcium in the circulation, is a not uncommon cause of death in women with breast cancer with massive bony metastases. Unfortunately, because the symptoms are often so equivocal the diagnosis may be missed. If a patient complains of malaise, fatigue, constipation, and thirst, the physician should carry out a serum calcium estimation. If hypercalcaemia is diagnosed, then urgent therapy is required. There are several techniques for getting hypercalcaemia under control, but in all cases a forced diuresis (excretion of urine) is required, supplemented by either corticosteroids, calcitonin, or phosphate therapy.

Orthopaedic problems

It is perhaps useful at this point to expand a little on the role of the orthopaedic surgeon, who may have to be consulted as part of a team dealing with advanced breast cancer. At post-mortem the skeleton is found to be involved in 75 per cent of women who have died of breast cancer. Bone pain or pathological fracture are a common presentation of the disease, and the breast primary may be overlooked for some time. If deposits in the femur (thigh bone) are present these may undergo pathological fracture in up to 50 per cent of cases, but the pathological fracture itself must not be considered a terminal event. (In the same way collapse of a dorsal vertebra, producing spinal cord compression, should be treated with the utmost urgency by removal of the lamina of the vertebra, because there is nothing more tragic than a woman spending her last 12 months confined to the wheelchair and incontinent of urine.) Pathological fractures of the femur demand operative internal fixation and there may even be a case for the fixation of large femoral deposits before they fracture. Pathological fractures of the humerus (in the upper arm) require non-operative fixation and in most cases treatment should be followed up by a short course of radiotherapy to the affected bone.

Progressive local or regional recurrence

I have left the problem of the local disease last on the list intentionally, as it leads naturally into the next section of this chapter. The local disease may include the original primary present at the time of detection of distant metastases, or may be represented by nodules or ulcers in the scar of a previous mastectomy, or by massive lymph node involvement in the underarm region on the same side, and above the collar-bone, often with extension of either skin or lymphatic deposits to the opposite side. As a sequel to massive underarm involvement secondary lymphoedema of the arm may develop, or alternatively pain and paralysis from infiltration of the network of nerves in the arm. In the majority

The advanced disease: palliation and terminal care

of cases such regional disease is not life-threatening, and it is conventional to judge the effectiveness of systemic therapy on the evidence of objective regression of the disease on the chest wall or within the regional lymph nodes. If the problem proves refractory to systemic treatment, then provided radiotherapy has not been previously used to maximum tolerated dose levels, this invaluable therapeutic weapon can again be called upon. Perhaps the most difficult and tragic of all the problems facing a woman dying of breast cancer is intractable lymphoedema of the arm. In spite of physiotherapy, elastic bandaging, and pneumatic compression therapy, a small minority of women may be left with the dreadful encumbrance of an immobile, grossly swollen arm. In these cases prevention is better than cure. Prevention is achieved by adequate local control of the disease at the time of primary therapy whilst bearing in mind that over-zealous therapy by combining radical surgery plus radiotherapy can itself produce the complication we wish to avoid.

Sequential systemic therapy

The sequence of therapy aimed at producing objective remission of the advanced disease and prolongation of the patient's life has evolved empirically and is often applied in a cookbook manner. It is for this reason that many doctors and nurses find the subject incredibly confusing. There are, however, conventional strategies for the treatment of premenopausal and postmenopausal women, and there is no doubt that by applying this kind of strategy many worthwhile and long-term remissions may be achieved. In the first instance simple endocrine therapy is favoured. For the premenopausal woman this would be surgical removal of the ovaries and for the postmenopausal woman additive endocrine agents with perhaps the anti-oestrogen Tamoxifen being the most effective and least toxic. In both pre- and postmenopausal women approximately a 30 per cent remission rate is to be expected.

95

Breast cancer: the facts

If there has been an unequivocal objective response to the first-line endocrine therapy, based on the objective measurements defined at the initial clinical evaluation of the patient, then on subsequent failure the patient may be considered for second-line endocrine therapy, either by surgery or further endocrine manipulation. Major endocrine ablation by removal of either the adrenal glands or the hypophysis was popular up to a few years ago, but the number of these operations being carried out in the United Kingdom is falling rapidly with improvement in the newer drugs. There is a natural reluctance to inflict such major procedures on a woman with a short expectation of life unless there are reasonable grounds to anticipate a good and prolonged response. These considerations have urged clinicians and biochemists to search for clues within the cancer itself that may predict whether or not the tumour is hormone dependent.

The oestradiol receptor

Target tissues that are sensitive to steroid hormones contain in the cytoplasm of their cells protein receptors that specifically bind and translocate the steroid to the nucleus (see Figure 3, page 23). Jensen in 1967 was the first to demonstrate that a cytoplasmic protein referred to as the oestradiol receptor ($E_2 R$) could be demonstrated in certain breast cancers. Following on this very important discovery many other workers have now demonstrated that if there is *no* detectable level of oestradiol receptor in the tumour, then endocrine therapy is unlikely to benefit the patient. Unfortunately, the converse is not true and even if there are high levels of oestradiol receptor detected in the tumour it still cannot be said with absolute certainty that the patient will respond. Nevertheless, using these and similar techniques, surgeons will soon be in the position to judge very accurately whether or not the patient is likely to benefit from endocrine ablative surgery. Although the initiative that led to the discovery of the $E_2 R$ related to the management of advanced breast cancer, it is likely that the most valuable contribution of this discovery will be in the scientific selection of the appropriate systemic therapy to be used following the treatment of primary carcinoma of the breast, as alluded to in Chapter 9.

Combination chemotherapy

As already mentioned, primary endocrine manoeuvres in patients with advanced breast cancer achieved remission rates of the order of 30 per cent. The use of single-agent cytotoxic therapy, for example with cyclophosphamide, produces a similar order of remission, perhaps at the cost of greater toxicity. In recent years the combination of three or more cytotoxic agents, each with different modes of action, with the drug combinations repeated at, say, monthly intervals, have produced far higher remission rates with some authorities claiming 80–90 per cent success. However, it must be emphasized that the 'success' is relative and merely refers to a temporary reduction in the tumour bulk at best lasting two years. This leaves unresolved the question of whether the inconvenience and unpleasantness of a monthly visit to the clinic for prescription and injection of toxic drugs is worth the increased chance of a temporary remission. For this reason it is still considered correct policy in the United Kingdom to adopt the soft option (simple endocrine therapy) first, and go on to combination chemotherapy only when this has failed. In the United States of America a different philosophy generally applies, in that most medical oncologists tend to favour the aggressive chemotherapy regimens, almost to the exclusion of endocrine manipulation. In all fairness, it must be emphasized that patients achieving a complete response on combination chemotherapy can enjoy a good quality of survival providing the signs and symptoms of the disease remit, but for those unfortunate patients who are failing on chemotherapy I believe it becomes an unacceptable additional burden to that imposed by the disease itself. Unfortunately, to date there is no accurate predictive test of response to cytotoxic therapy as has been developed for endocrine therapy.

Terminal care

It is difficult to define precisely what we mean by terminal care. Probably this phase of management of a patient with breast cancer is entered once active therapy aimed at prolongation of life is abandoned in favour of palliation alone. Even so such patients might survive between a few days or a couple of years, such is the unpredictable nature of the disease. For this reason it is also very difficult to judge whether the remaining period of life should be spent at home, in a hospital, or in a hospice for the dying. One feels instinctively that a patient should end her days in the bosom of her family, amongst close friends and familiar objects; yet a hospice for the dying provides the most expert medical and nursing care and at the same time spares the immediate family, who might be very distressed by coping with the needs of a dying relative. Some sort of compromise is probably ideal, in which the patient is admitted initially to a hospice, where symptoms are carefully defined and treatment prescribed, and once she is in a relatively stable condition on the correct schedule of drugs, she returns home to her family with follow-up care from either a domiciliary team or the family practitioner. Thereafter, should her condition change and the symptoms once more become out of control, a further admission for stabilization could be arranged. Unfortunately, in many countries this aspect of care in the community is very badly organized at present, so that many dying women suffer needlessly.

The needs of the dying patient can be divided up into spiritual and physical. I am not equipped or trained to comment on the spiritual needs of the dying, but a religious person should be allowed the peace of mind provided by prayer and allowed every opportunity of visits by the clergy. At the same time, one should respect the wishes of the unbelievers in the community as it can be distressing for some patients to have unwelcome visits from well-meaning priests.

In the previous section I dealt in some detail with symptomatic control. The problems of pain, anxiety, and insomnia are very badly handled by members of the medical profession and yet we have sufficient drugs within our armamentarium to deal with all these problems in a way that would control the symptoms without blunting the intellect. The problem is usually one of inadequate prescription rather than over-prescribing. Brompton's mixture, containing morphia in a suspension medium containing alcohol, can be prescribed in doses titrated to control the pain, with the frequency of the dose being manoeuvred in such a way that the patient never experiences pain and never needs to beg for the next dose. The problems of addiction seldom arise and the total dose of drugs given is lower than if analgesics are given only on demand. Some patients with liver secondaries have considerable nausea, which could be aggravated by Brompton's mixture, and in these cases the addition of Largactil may be appropriate.

I would never advocate euthanesia, which must be a counsel of therapeutic bankruptcy. With skilled medical and nursing care, life should be tolerable even in the face of the worst ravages that can be inflicted by carcinoma of the breast.

Conclusion

The management of women with advanced breast cancer is becoming increasingly complicated and demands close collaboration between surgeon, radiotherapist, medical oncologist and, if possible, the hospice team. Ideally, therefore, these patients should be treated in combined multidisciplinary clinics. The sequencing of systemic therapy is probably of less importance than the practice of good medicine by proper evaluation of the patient on presentation and the provision

of adequate symptomatic control. It is also of greatest importance to judge when further active therapy is no longer indicated so that the patient may be allowed to die with dignity
and comfort.

13

The future

For the purpose of discussion, I would like to divide up the future into the current decade 1980–9, the next decade, 1990–2000, and possible developments from the year 2001. In the next decade I foresee steady progress along current established lines of research and development. In the last decade of this century I can foresee the realization of promising new developments that I have hinted at in this book, whereas for the twenty-first century my extrapolations become science fiction.

Present–1989

In the next few years I think that we can confidently anticipate that the questions concerning screening, breast conservation, and adjuvant systemic therapy will be answered once and for all. As far as screening is concerned, forgetting my natural scepticism, I would sincerely hope that a high-risk population can be readily defined and that cost-effective ways of diagnosing breast cancer before its dissemination can be evolved that will ultimately lead to an overall reduction in mortality from breast cancer. By the very nature of the disease, which can disseminate long before it is detectable by any known methodology, I would predict that only modest improvements can be anticipated by this approach.

As far as breast conservation is concerned, here the problem is of a different order. We are not interested in determining whether breast conservation actually improves the survival following the treatment of primary breast cancer; what we really need to know is whether conservative measures are equivalent to mastectomy as far as local control of the disease is concerned as well as life salvage. Statistically, this is a much harder nut to crack, but at the very best we can hope that current and anticipated trials of breast conservation will at least allow us accurately to define the risk to the patient of conserving the breast, so that she will be able to make an informed rather than emotional judgement as to whether the risk of conserving the breast is acceptable or not. Only when these hard data are available can we reasonably ask the patient herself to make a value judgement, which to date has been based on over-interpretation of uncontrolled studies overlaid with a healthy dose of wishful thinking.

The most confident prediction that I can make for the next decade concerns the role of adjuvant systemic therapy. At the moment I think it is still an open question whether the addition of cytotoxic or endocrine therapy following adequate local treatment will prolong life in addition to delaying the appearance of recurrence. A sufficient number of well-designed prospective controlled trials are in progress around the world at the moment to answer these questions with a high degree of confidence by the end of the decade. Again, I do not share the excessive optimism of some of my colleagues about this approach and, again, I would predict modest gains prolonging survival in perhaps 10–20 per cent more women with early breast cancer. Nevertheless, because the disease is so common even these modest gains will be reflected in the thousands of women who will live these added years that will see their children through school or see the birth of their grandchildren. In parallel with these studies it is likely that early progress will be made along the lines of being able to select the appropriate systemic arm of treatment based on the biological characteristics of the individual cancer.

As far as the woman with recurrent or advanced breast cancer is concerned, I can foresee little cause for optimism. At best we can aim to prolong life at minimal cost in terms of suffering by employing agents of less toxicity than those currently available and by developing new techniques of symptomatic palliation.

The future

1990–2000

In twenty years' time I anticipate, with a lesser degree of confidence, the realization of some promising new developments and ideas. I think it is likely that we shall be well along the road to defining the aetiological factors in the induction of breast cancer, and at the same time be in the position to commence trials of prevention. I also anticipate the development of a biochemical test on blood samples that would allow the early detection of breast cancer at its curable stage.

With the established primary cancer I predict that laboratory tests will become available that will identify accurately the behaviour of the disease, the extent of its dissemination, and the systemic therapy most likely to be appropriate. In addition, I think a 'tumour marker' will appear that will allow us accurately to monitor the amount of residual tumour at any time following the primary treatment, so as to modulate in type or dose the systemic therapy required. Using established agents systemically, but guided and aided by the ideal tumour marker, a more important impact on survival for early breast cancer than blind systemic therapy will become apparent. Again, using the same approach, patients with recurrent or advanced breast cancer might experience significant prolongation of life, so that we can begin to talk about 'cures' in what at the moment are the least promising subjects.

The new century

I suppose if any scientist was asked to predict a major advance for the year 2000 in the management of breast cancer, the natural response would be to suggest a new type of drug based on a better understanding of the malignant transformation. This might be an agent related to interferon with its unique biological properties, although I must hasten to emphasize that at this juncture there is no good evidence that interferon itself has any unique effect on breast cancer that could not

103

be achieved at much less expense by a conventional cytotoxic chemotherapy.

To my own taste this approach, however sophisticated, indicates tunnel vision. Science is a continuous process of approximation to the truth and no single generation is ever gifted with the insight to solve a problem in its entirety. Thus, Newtonian physics and the Darwinian theory of evolution went a long way to explaining many of the observed phenomena of the physical world and the biosphere. Their theories have been modified and to some extent overtaken by Einsteinian physics and the newer schools of thought on evolution following the revolutionary discovery of the mechanisms of genetic coding. Thus it is likely to be with breast cancer. The contemporary theory that the outcome of treatment is predetermined by the extent of micro-metastases at the time of diagnosis, and that the metastases arise from cells shed from the primary tumour along venous pathways early in its evolution, may only be part of the truth. Certainly this theory is more attractive than the classical mechanistic approach of dissemination via the lymphatic system described by Halsted. The new hypothesis must also be considered fertile in that it has generated new therapeutic approaches which in their turn have led to the promise of prolonging survival of the disease. Nonetheless, I would predict again with confidence that our generation has been gifted with less than a complete insight into the problem. It makes an attractive parlour game to come up with alternative hypotheses, however whimsical, that might conceivably provide a more complete explanation of the observed phenomena in the treatment of breast cancer. For example, I have heard the idea expressed that metastases do not in fact arise from intact cells capable of cloning but might conceivably result from 'infection' of the target tissue with genetic material shed by the cancer cells. This foreign DNA might, for example, code a normal liver cell to express the morphological and growth characteristics of a breast cancer cell. Although this may sound very far-fetched indeed, surely such a mechanism would go some way towards explaining why some tissues such as the liver and bone marrow are common sites for secondary growth, whereas the muscles of the body almost never harbour secondaries.

Ignoring the previous example, I hope it can be appreciated why it is essential for clinicians and scientists to keep an open mind at all times, acknowledge new data as new facts when corroborated by the scientific method, and not to be disappointed if these new facts fail to confirm their previously cherished beliefs, but to build them into new hypotheses which can be tested in their own turn. I freely acknowledge that these philosophical ramblings are merely a facile distillation of the works of Carl Popper, but if we are not to repeat the mistakes of the last one hundred years by rigid adherence to an obsolete concept of the disease, then some detached vision of reality is mandatory.

The inhibition of progress

In this final chapter I have tried to define the basis for reasonable optimism concerning the treatment of breast cancer, but there are a number of factors that could inhibit progress. The cancer researchers' perpetual cry for more money and the complaints about the lack of resources are probably the least important. Left alone with the current resources available, clinicians and basic scientists have the wherewithal to make the progress that I have outlined. My real fear is that a flight from rationalism will ruin the chances of real progress. I have already pointed out how the doctors themselves could be guilty of translating reasonable new theories into a new dogma which could inhibit progress in the same way that the rigid adherence to Halsted's teachings have done over the last century. Already I can see this creeping in as clinicians, particularly in America, claim that adjuvant chemotherapy is already of proven benefit and that it works because it *should* work. This is in many ways analogous to the attitudes of the surgeons at the turn of the century who stated that radical mastectomy was the treatment of choice because it was the only way of removing all the disease. These individuals have been succinctly described by Dr. Bernard Fisher as having 'one foot in Halsted's grave and one foot in outer space'.

There are also disturbing signs of flight from rationalism on the part of the patients. This is partly tied up with the mood of anti-professionalism and partly a spin-off from some of the cults of the West Coast of America. In my Preface, I described how the anti-professional stance of the feminist lobby had led to the therapeutic anarchy that exists in some parts of America. In what other branch of medicine does the patient demand to make the decisions? I can only repeat my plea that women should trust the medical profession, that they are working for the benefit of womankind, as once this trust is lost there is no hope at all. You might just as well put yourself in the hands of the herbalists or other fringe practitioners.

One of the greatest tragedies that I encounter in the treatment of patients with breast cancer is in the connection with the practice of fringe medicine. Somewhere in the world there are always unscrupulous individuals who will trade off the despair of the dying. It never ceases to amaze me that otherwise rational and intelligent human beings can believe that a magic cure is available in California or in the Bavarian Alps providing you have sufficient funds available. This leads on many occasions to desperate husbands and families selling up all their worldly goods to purchase the miraculous cure. The unscrupulous practitioners on the fringe often portray themselves as victims of the medical establishment and yet they prosper wonderfully as a result of their uncritical prescription of diets, purges, mud baths, and herbal extracts. If the patient dies they always have their cry: 'if only she had come earlier'; if the woman lives another two or three years they claim success, whereas the unpredictable natural history of the disease would account for any of the successes claimed by the fringe. 'Conventional medicine' is sometimes used as a per-

The future

jorative term, yet if I were to try and define the distinction between the mainstream and the fringe, it would be concerned with the degree of self-criticism. I feel that doctors are essentially humble. We recognize our deficiencies and discuss them freely amongst ourselves. Naturally, in order to inspire some degree of confidence amongst our patients we have to apply a veneer of self-confidence, which may not always be felt. In contrast, the practitioners on the fringe have divine insight that their eccentric methods are the only way to cure cancer and would never acknowledge that the patient lives in spite of the treatment rather than because of it.

Providing we resist this flight from rationalism into a new Dark Age of therapeutic insanity, and in spite of the world-wide recession which threatens the budget of most research institutions, I am truly optimistic that we will establish more and more facts concerning the nature of breast cancer, so that by the end of the century the disease will cease to be a scourge and if nothing else the second edition of this book will be fatter and more optimistic.

Index

Index

radiation
   ionizing 13, 38
   radiotherapy 58, 59, 62, 89, 91, 93
      postoperative 64–6
      side effects 65–6
   X-rays 13, 38
radiotherapy 58, 59, 62, 89, 91, 93
   postoperative 64–6
   side effects 65–6
reactive hyperplasia 35
recurrence 65, 79, 94–5
rehabilitation 76–80
remission 95, 97
risk factors 7–14
   breast-feeding 8–10
   age at first pregnancy 8, 9–10
   menstruation 10
   contraceptive pill 10–11
   HRT 11
   genetic factors 12
   viruses 12
   ionizing radiation 13, 38

sampling the tumour 44–7, 61
sarcomata 30
scirrhous cancer, *see* invasive duct cancer
Scotland 9
screening 36–40, 72–3, 101
secondary diseases 35
self-examination 39–40, *Plate 1*, 72–3
sexual problems 77–8
silicone implants 61
size of tumour 32, 36, 40, 54
spread of disease in the body, *see* metastasis
stages of breast cancer 5–6, 53, 54, 60, 89
structure of breast 15–24
subcutaneous mastectomy 61

supernumerary breasts 15, 27, 28
surgery 20, 55–63
survival, rate of, *see* prognosis
Sweden 9
Syme, James 3
symptoms 25–35, 41–7, 92, 93

Tamoxifen 68, 95
terminal care 98–100
Thailand 9
thermography 46
treatment
   chemotherapy 68–70, 97–8
      side effects 69
   endocrine therapy 67–8, 95–6
   radiotherapy 58, 59, 62, 89, 91, 93
      postoperative 64–6
      side effects 65–6
   surgery 20, 55–63
   see also palliation; terminal care
tuberculosis 27
tumours
   benign 11, 24, 25–6, 26–9
   definition 26
   malignant 26, 30–5
   size of 32, 36, 40, 54

UICC 53, 54
UK 1, 8, 9, 10, 11, 38, 60, 62, 68, 76, 97
ulceration of skin 4, 32, 49
ultrasonography 46
USA 1, 7, 9, 11, 36–7, 62, 69, 97

Vesalius 2
viruses, transmission by 12

X-rays 13, 38

Yugoslavia 9